T0304936

'This dynamic book draws upon the perspec[tive...] people and highly experienced and creative voice practitioners to present a philosophically original, practical and integrated approach to voice and communication work. It is psychologically challenging in the best possible ways and highlights how deeper levels of reflexivity on the part of therapists and clients can overcome subconscious biases that may influence or limit our approaches to this important work. It is refreshing in its inclusion of so many different voices, and has prompted me to think differently about how I would now enter this therapeutic space.'

– *Janet Baker, LACST, MSc, PhD, Clinical Member ITAA and family therapist, author of* Psychosocial Perspectives on the Management of Voice Disorders

'This book is required reading for all practitioners who work at the complex intersection of voice, gender and identity. Based on vivid and extensive documentation of the lived experience, it provides insightful and exceptional understanding, together with clear practical approaches. Both radical in its inclusivity and heroic in its challenge, it is a vital text for all those who endorse the right to vocal autonomy.'

– *Jane Boston, Leader MA/MFA Voice Studies: Teaching and Coaching, The Royal Central School of Speech and Drama, London*

'Coming out as one's true self, and speaking in a voice which we feel is intrinsically our own, are acts of protest, courage and resilience. This book indeed goes beyond a training guide for voice teachers, therapists and gender specialists. This is a book about identity and social justice, it champions collaboration with the community and makes explicit the power dynamics in the clinical context.'

– *Lord Michael Cashman, Founder of Stonewall, author of* One of Them: From Albert Square to Parliament Square

'Complementing their previous self-help book for trans people, the same authors have now turned their attention to helping speech and language therapists develop their own skills too, harnessing a wide range of expert knowledge. I had always imagined SLT to be a discipline mainly focused on technique and exercise. What I got from this book, above all, was an understanding that it is a far more holistic process, reaching into the psychological domain and framing identity as the foundation of vocal presentation.'

– *Christine Burns, MBE, author and transgender activist*

Voice and Communication Therapy with Trans and Non-Binary People

Sharing the Clinical Space

Matthew Mills and **Gillie Stoneham**

Forewords by Meg-John Barker and
Elizabeth van Horn

Illustrated by Charlotte Retief

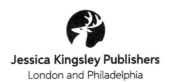

Jessica Kingsley Publishers
London and Philadelphia

First published in 2021
by Jessica Kingsley Publishers
73 Collier Street
London N1 9BE, UK

www.jkp.com

Library of Congress Cataloging in Publication Data
A CIP catalog record for this book is available from the Library of Congress

British Library Cataloguing in Publication Data
A CIP catalogue record for this book is available from the British Library

ISBN 978 1 78775 104 0
eISBN 978 1 78775 105 7

Printed and bound in Great Britain

Contents

Contents

Foreword

MEG-JOHN BARKER

Matthew Mills and Gillie Stoneham's *Voice and Communication Therapy with Trans and Non-Binary People: Sharing the Clinical Space* is a follow-up to their excellent *The Voice Book for Trans and Non-Binary People*, but this time aimed at practitioners rather than trans and non-binary people looking to engage with their voices themselves.

On the face of it this may seem like quite a specialist book for speech and language therapists and voice practitioners focused on working with trans people. However, there is much rich and helpful material in here for all practitioners and therapists working with clients across gender diversity. It becomes clear that the process of finding your voice – in a literal sense – is intrinsically linked to the existential voice-finding and narrative story-telling which is a vital part of healing and growth for all of us. Also the mindful, embodied, process-focused rather than goal-focused approach to voice-finding is usefully applicable to many other areas of therapy and life more widely. Finally, the reflective, intersectional, compassion-focused perspective taken by the authors throughout is one which all practitioners working across difference would benefit from.

Reading the book feels like attending a well-facilitated workshop where we learn about all aspects of supporting people – psychologically and practically – through doing this work. The views and experiences of practitioners and clients are constantly woven in to bring the material to life, and to give an ongoing sense of the diversity of desires and practices in this area. I also appreciated the recognition of the paradox throughout the book around 'for whom and for what purpose change is sought and desired'. Mills and Stoneham capture the complexity for trans and non-binary people of holding both the desire for authenticity and the yearning for belonging in a culture which still understands gender in simplistic, static, binary ways.

I was particularly struck, throughout the book, by the commitment shown by the authors to be effective allies working in a culturally competent way to create a therapeutic alliance with trans and non-binary people, and helping others to do so as well. At a time when we are in the midst of a trans moral panic, and so many of us are silenced, this book does much to give a literal and metaphorical voice to trans community as equal and alongside cis allies. This is in stark opposition to the othering or saviour-style approaches that are prevalent in wider culture and sadly still among some practitioners. There is indeed much to learn from here.

Dr Meg-John Barker is a writer, senior lecturer, psychotherapist and co-author of *Gender: A Graphic Guide* and *How to Understand Your Gender* and co-editor of *Genderqueer and Non-Binary Genders*

Foreword

Elizabeth van Horn

The title of this book suggests that the authors are primarily targeting speech and language therapy and voice professionals in giving a guide to how to deliver voice and communication therapy to people who identify as transgender or non-binary. However, I would suggest that this book will appeal to a much wider audience. It will potentially be of benefit to any professional working with this diverse group, whether they be operating in specialist gender identity services or other more generic health and social care settings. It strikes me as unashamedly and refreshingly political, not shying away from the reality that trans and non-binary people have been historically misunderstood and marginalized and many continue to experience this. It is refreshing to read a text which acknowledges this, since this is the only way that delivering good care can really be achieved – by acknowledging and confronting our realities.

This book offers a unique opportunity for those of us seeking to deliver effective and quality care to our patients, but, in so doing, invites us to not only think about the challenges that those seeking help from us face, but also pushes us to challenge ourselves, to be open to thinking more broadly and more personally, to reflect on the impact of our culture, and family experiences, our preconceptions and prejudices, and to explore how our own gender identity has and continues to impact on our lives. It emphasizes that we all have some form of gender identity (including those identifying as agender), and the importance of acknowledging that we can learn as much from our patients as they can learn from us, with the goal that, by engaging in this way, we will be better able to understand what it feels like to be trans or non-binary in a polarized society, where individuals are labelled, judged and ultimately often experience, at best, marginalization, and at worst are excluded.

There is a huge amount of honesty in this book about the difficulties in overcoming challenges faced, but also an encouraging and not unrealistic sense of positivity, demonstrating that things can get better and that with the right support, those identifying as trans and non-binary can be helped, if help is sought. This is illustrated by the many generous and honest personal examples of those with both professional expertise and those with lived expertise. For me, the main message was that collectively we can all strive to move forward as a society to help people get to a better place where they feel not only happier with their voice, but that they are assisted in really developing a *voice*, such that they are not only more at ease with themselves but empowered to feel more confident and productive in a holistic sense, which of course has not only personal benefit, but wider benefit since healthier and happier individuals are able to function more effectively and contribute more, and that of course advantages all of us.

The authors have chosen a very accessible format to present their ideas, which draws the reader in and this book is extremely easy to read. It is formatted in five chapters, with the first orientating the reader to the 'task in hand'. Text is frequently followed by exercises encouraging the reader to take some time to reflect on what they have learnt. There are also numerous illustrative diagrams, along with fascinating narratives. It feels almost like it has a 'handbook' or 'instruction manual' quality in that the academic content of the text is consistently linked to and reminds us that we are reading this not simply to gain knowledge but to *apply* what we have learnt for the benefit of our clients. The frequent clinical vignettes, and stories of real lived experience, along with often very open comments from professionals, all of which help to make this book 'come alive', and my experience was of reading something, not dry, crusty and removed, but of gaining knowledge whilst always having the personal in mind. Specific sections focus on different 'spaces' (although many of the themes bridge these spaces) including the gender, the psychological, the vocal and the social space and lastly, the _____ space, the latter again inviting the reader to think for themselves and choose their own name for this section of the text.

In conclusion, this book is both informative but also very moving, and because of the narrative style and multiple examples of individuals' unique and shared experiences, demonstrates the many complex and varied journeys that many of trans and non-binary identifying people are taking, which we as professionals are privileged to share through our clinical contact. This includes experiences of disaffection and indifference but also of fortitude, friendship, progress and creativity.

I found this book informative, thought-provoking and uplifting. I was put in touch with the sense of collective purpose, which as clinicians I think we can all easily lose touch with intermittently in the melee of day-to-day clinical work, sometimes leaving us more focused on paperwork than people. It seemed appropriate to me to end with a quote from Octavio Paz's *Labyrinth of Silence* (1967):

> What sets worlds in motion is the interplay of differences, their attractions and repulsions. Life is plurality, death is uniformity. By suppressing differences and peculiarities, by eliminating different civilizations and cultures, progress weakens life and favours death. The ideal of a single civilization for everyone, implicit in the cult of progress and technique, impoverishes and mutilates us. Every view of the world that becomes extinct, every culture that disappears, diminishes a possibility of life.

His views, I suspect, will be in harmony with both authors and I hope will resonate with any reader of this book.

Dr Elizabeth van Horn is a Consultant Psychiatrist in Gender Dysphoria at the 'Charing Cross' Gender Identity Clinic, Tavistock & Portman NHS Foundation Trust

Acknowledgements

The contributors gave permission to be credited exactly as listed, and described themselves as follows.

KEY FOR CONTRIBUTORS:

Art Psychotherapist (AP)

Expert by Experience (E) (trans and non-binary people)

Musician (M)

Partner (P)

Psychologist (Psy)

Speech and Language Therapist (SLT)

Voice Coach (V)

Medical Doctor (MD)

Barbara Aster (E) wife of Jenny – partners for 35 years; former boxer; now a housewife and cook; trans awareness trainer for Metropolitan Police; advocates for social justice.

Jenny Aster (P) wife of Barbara – partners for 35 years; she works in university student counselling and mental health; advocates for social justice.

Pippa Baker (E) attended voice therapy and a voice group; someone who happens to stammer and embraces it; red hot 6'1" business woman.

Stephanie Bales (E) attended voice therapy and a voice group; her philosophy: 'If someone throws the ball, catch it and run, then paint it pink!'

Jenny-Anne Bishop OBE (E) attended voice therapy; she is a campaigner and community supporter.

Carys Bracken (SLT) Advanced Speech and Language Therapist at the 'Charing Cross' Gender Identity Clinic, Tavistock & Portman NHS Foundation Trust.

Sara Belinda Brown (E) attended therapy and a voice group; writer; in the sisterhood.

Stephen Davidson (E, M) is an improvised theatre practitioner, author, choir leader and trans activist.

Skye Davies (E, Psy) is a non-binary person working as an Assistant Psychologist in the NHS. They are interested in the application of community psychology principles to trans healthcare.

Lucy Dyer (E, M) attended voice therapy and a voice group; musician and actress.

Jenny Etherington (E) attended voice therapy and a voice group; she has *the* shoes, she has *the* car; her slogan: 'One life, live it!'

Sarah F (E) attended voice therapy and a voice group.

Gwen Ford (E) attended voice therapy and a voice group; she is a level 12 Warlock and vows not to use her vocal training for evil.

Jennifer Foreman (E) attended voice therapy and a voice group; business woman.

Ioanna Georgiadou (SLT) Highly Specialist Speech and Language Therapist at the Nottingham Centre for Transgender Health; voice and communication member of scientific committee for European Association of Transgender Health (EPATH).

Linda Glover (E) attended voice therapy and a voice group.

Nicky Gorb (SLT) Advanced Speech and Language Therapist at the 'Charing Cross' Gender Identity Clinic, Tavistock & Portman NHS Foundation Trust.

Danielle Hewett (E) attended voice therapy and a voice group; navigator and survivor of the 'rapids' and currents in the river of life.

Kaidyn Hinds (E, M) attended voice therapy and a voice group; professional singer and actor.

Mia Hughes (E, M) attended voice therapy and a voice group; singer-songwriter, punk band frontwoman and part-time tutor.

Luna Johns (E) swore her way through voice therapy and a voice group.

Nazlin Kurji-Smith (SLT) Chair of Trans and Non-Binary Voice and

Communication National Clinical Excellence Network of Royal College of Speech and Language Therapists, Lead Speech and Language Therapist at the Northern Region Dysphoria Service.

Jan Logan (SLT) is a specialist speech and language therapist, counsellor and narrative therapist.

LPT (E) attended voice therapy and a voice group.

Leah Lynch (E) attended voice therapy and a voice group.

Amanda Malovics (E) attended voice therapy and a voice group; she left behind her own country to build herself up in another one.

Justine Mole (E) attended voice therapy and a voice group.

Barbara Molteno (SLT) Lead Specialist Speech and Language Therapist at the Porterbrook Gender Clinic, Sheffield.

Mary Moos (SLT) Specialist Speech and Language Therapist at the 'Charing Cross' Gender Identity Clinic, Tavistock & Portman NHS Foundation Trust.

Annie Morrison (V) is a voice coach at the Royal Academy of Dramatic Art; originally a speech and language therapist specializing in voice.

Sasha Myerson (E) attended voice therapy and a voice group; she is a PhD student at Birkbeck College (University of London).

Kate Nambiar (E, MD) is a Specialty Doctor in Sexual Health and HIV Medicine in Brighton, and a Specialty Doctor in Gender Identity Medicine at the 'Charing Cross' Gender Identity Clinic, Tavistock & Portman NHS Foundation Trust.

Catherine O'Neill (AP, SLT) is a specialist speech and language therapist, art psychotherapist and a registered intermediary.

Nadine Osborne (E) attended voice therapy.

Anny Parnell (SLT) is a speech and language therapist in training.

Nina Perez (E) attended voice therapy; expert by experience panellist in the NHS, scrutineer and council member of the British Association of Gender Identity Specialists.

Sean Pert (SLT) Specialist Advisor for the Royal College of Speech and Language Therapists; Senior Clinical Lecturer at University of Manchester; Vice Chair of RCSLT Trans Voice and Communication Clinical Excellence Network; trans voice speech and language therapist at LGBT Foundation, Manchester.

Rachel Preston (SLT) is a speech and language therapist in training.

Indigo Jonah Raphael (E) attended voice therapy; having been a Congregational

Rabbi, he now works as Chaplain in an NHS Chaplaincy-Spiritual Care Team. He is Trans and Non-Binary Rep on the LGBT+ and Friends Staff Network in his Trust; he is husband of Ruthie.

Ruthie Raphael (P) previously worked in the city and as a volunteer counsellor; now a professional dog groomer. She embraces her own non-binary view of gender. Ruthie is wife of Indigo and together they celebrate their Queer identities.

Rebecca (E) attended voice therapy and a voice group.

Christina Riley (E) attended voice therapy; an out-and-proud trans model in the construction and engineering sector, advocate and public speaker on LGBTQ+ inclusion in workplace, receiver of LGBT Awards Corporate Rising Star award 2017 and Inclusive Company highly recommended 2018.

Sophie Russell (E) attended voice therapy and a voice group; totally trans trucker.

Dee Ryder (E) attended voice therapy and a voice group; film producer.

Natasha Stavropoulos (E, Psy) attended voice therapy; she is a Greek-British sex work-positive, openly trans psychologist and addictions counsellor.

SB (E) attended voice therapy and a voice group.

Zoe Smallwood (E) is a software engineer from Cambridge who attended the voice therapy and voice group.

Daniella Stewart (E) attended voice therapy and a voice group; lover of life and people.

Maggi Stratford (V) is a voice coach at Leeds Gender Clinic; psychotherapist.

James Sunderland (E) attended voice therapy and a voice group.

Erin Sutton (E) attended voice therapy and a voice group.

Sophie Thurston (E) attended voice therapy and a voice group; 38 years old and trying to give herself the best chance at her transition.

Scarlett Heaven Worraker (E) attended voice therapy and a voice group; music lover; trend-setter.

Thanks to the following who offered *additional* editorial, technical, supervisory and peer review input: Dr James Barrett, Carys Bracken, Emily Bruni, Sally Collins, Dr Vanessa Crawford, Skye Davies, Nick Drake, Simon Anthony Ford, Nicola Gorb, Dr Helen Greener, Mark Hayward, Jan Logan, Pam Milman, Mary Moos, Annie Morrison, Dr Kate Nambiar, Jeannette Nelson, Catherine O'Neill, Valerie Peden, Philip Robinson, John Stack, Annie Tunnicliffe and Dr Ben Vincent.

Introduction

WHY THIS BOOK?

Our first book, *The Voice Book for Trans and Non-Binary People*, was primarily written for, and in collaboration with, the trans community. It provides a practical voice guide for those wishing to develop voice and communication skills. As it happens, the book has also been well received by voice professionals, both in terms of our own written perspective, and that of the many experts by experience who contributed. This companion book is not a rewriting of what has gone before. Our aim here is to invite a broader exploration of trans and non-binary cultural competence, and a deeper engagement with vocal process and trans affirmative practice.

This book celebrates a community of voices and perspectives that speak to the fundamentals of this collaboration. We affirm people and join them in celebrating their sense of self. Whilst we hope this book examines some of the complexities in the field, we encourage you, the reader, simply to bring your humanity and meet the client where they are.

The book takes a narrative and practical approach which centres the expertise of people in their lives. It brings together practical exercises, client wisdom, clinical and practitioner experience, and an overview of theory. We refer the reader elsewhere for aspects of medical, surgical and legal issues. Our philosophy is multi-dimensional: primarily we need to develop trans awareness, and to understand our role in facilitating vocal change; we also need to understand the intersections of gender and privilege with our clients. As part of this, we need to dive deeply into more understanding of our own voices in order to demonstrate and coach others; finally, we need to know group process and the value of community support, witnessing and sharing. From examining ourselves as helpers, and developing our own affirmative positionality, new stories are encouraged that open us to working towards our own redundancy.

The structure of this book follows our philosophy, with each chapter describing pertinent 'spaces' in the work:

- Gender: the information, themes and discussion were shaped principally by the trans and non-binary people, clinicians and clients, whom we interviewed.

- Psychological: we examine the role we take in therapeutic alliance and the psychological approaches we favour, illustrated by client comment and documentation.

- Vocal: we invite the reader to be both a vocal explorer and vocal coach, with particular attention to relational practice.

- Social: we explore group process and how we hold the space differently in building community of support.

- Emerging space: we end with an anthology of stories and journeys of resilience so that, having heard them, you may be moved to transform your own personal and working spaces.

We will look back on this moment of human history as a time of re-examining human and systemic identity statements, of acknowledging our global humanity and shared fragility. On the one hand, we are increasingly able to embrace a diverse range of human self-expression; on the other, in a binary construction, the global, political and social landscapes have become more violent, oppositional and fragmented. The antidote is sharing resources, developing compassion and growing community.

We are human. Our response to a set of circumstances is a function of our perception. As we are learning to share, so we are holding labels and boundaries more wisely so that we can both respect people's self-identifications and also hold our own without feeling challenged. We encourage the reader to hold their sense of community and possibility as they listen to the many voices in this book: transformational voices that call out in celebration of diversity and compassion.

We are grateful to all the contributors in this book who gave their time and expertise, and whose openness and honesty showed courage and generosity.

WHO ARE WE?

We write from both a collaborative and an individual space. Synchronous perspectives that we hold about our trans voice and communication work have driven the desire to share this with the wider voice practitioner community. In doing so, we are learning more about what it is to live as humans in relationship to each other. Our individual experiencing means that we have travelled to this point differently, and in this process we are each other's teachers, supervisors and support. Here is a little of what we bring to this book:

Matthew is cisgender (he/him) and trained and worked as a professional actor, singer and pianist for many years before becoming a speech and language therapist. He is a gay rights campaigner, HIV survivor, and activist. He is a consultant speech and language therapist at the 'Charing Cross' Gender Identity Clinic, where he heads the voice and communication service. He is current President of the British Association of Gender Identity Specialists and external examiner at Royal Central School of Speech and Drama (voice studies). He brings a deep commitment to social justice, personal authenticity and compassionate service to the heart of therapeutic work.

Gillie is cisgender (she/her) and brings many years' experience as a facilitator, coach, counsellor and specialist speech and language therapist. She has a consultancy in voice and personal impact and works as a specialist trans voice therapist in the 'Charing Cross' Gender Identity Clinic. Her many years' experience as a senior lecturer in speech and language therapy have focused on personal and professional communication and leadership, in addition to voice. In this work, she brings a passion for facilitating the exploration of creative ways of being with clients, and being within the therapeutic space, which deconstruct notions of collaboration and holism.

The process that we have between us is unique and fruitful. Writing this book has involved the surfacing of deep and honest reflections and also the celebrating of struggle, in order to voice our collective thoughts as written text for others to read. We stay open to the vulnerability of sharing our voice, in the way that our contributors are also sharing so generously. What emerges from the work fosters tacit knowledge that changes us as people in our wider communities – truly a gestalt.

CHAPTER 1

The Gender Space

—— TOWARDS EFFECTIVE ALLYSHIP ——

THIS CHAPTER WILL ASK

What attitudes, behaviours and practices foster cultural sensitivity and enable us to reclaim our ideology and work affirmatively?

How can we build reflexive, respectful communities in our work together?

CULTURAL COMPETENCE

Cultural competence is the ability to understand, interact and communicate effectively with people across diverse cultures. It is not simply about respecting the context of people's lives, but, within healthcare, encompasses the delivery of evidence-based care that is ethical, sensitive and person-centred. Betancourt *et al.* (2003) summarize this as 'the ability of systems to provide care to patients with diverse values, beliefs and behaviours, including tailoring delivery to meet patients' social, cultural, and linguistic needs' (p.v). Kirmayer (2012) cites evidence that attention to these factors can reduce health disparities. This chapter aims to set out the fundamentals of being culturally competent to work with trans and non-binary people in exploring voice and communication. It examines concepts for establishing and developing trans affirmative, transparent and responsible practice. *Quis custodiet ipsos custodies* (Juvenal, Satires VI 347–348) is the maxim 'who watches the watchers/who will guard the guards themselves?' and speaks of the accountability required of those who have and hold power (see Richards *et al.*, 2014). Increasing our knowledge and engaging in reflexive practice are the two essential ingredients that underpin affirmative ways of being. We affirm difference by recognizing our own relation to difference, our own gender identity and how we perform it in relation to normative expectations. In so doing, we move beyond the potential patronage of simply being accepting of others, and embrace the dynamic, lifelong process of developing cultural humility (Tervalon and Murray-Garcia, 1998). Reflexivity partners accountability. Developing awareness and taking committed action beat at the heart of this book – enabling the facilitation of safe, respectful and deeply examined clinical and pedagogical practice. Feminist, poet and civil rights activist, Audre Lorde wrote that 'revolution is not a one-time event. It is becoming always vigilant for the smallest opportunity to make a genuine change in established, outgrown responses' (1984/2019, pp.135–6). Seeking, understanding and negotiating meaning is never ending (do Mar Pereira, 2017).

> Every person – regardless of intellect or training – is a product of their social environment, and so even the most well-intentioned person can internalise and uncritically reproduce behaviour and beliefs that are potentially problematic or harmful. Reflexive practice can minimise this. (Vincent, 2018, p.40)

Jenny-Anne (E): It's really important that speech and language therapists have both voice skills and also psychological awareness skills, therapeutic skills, so that they have an empathy with trans people, and an understanding of the huge spectrum of gender diversity, and that some people want to be identified within the male–female binary, and others don't, they want to be identified outside that, or between, or some people are even playful with gender – that they really don't want you to know!

WHAT UNITES US

To be human is to be complex – we know it and we live it. We deeply desire to belong and we long to be desirable to others. We strive to claim our space and set boundaries, yet hope to be accepted – seen and heard as who we know and perceive ourselves to be. The evolution of the human brain poses challenges to integrate threat, drive and soothing responses (Gilbert, 2015; Irons, 2019) (for more on this see Chapter 2). Sharing is fundamental but has to be learned and balanced with self-protection. This is the very process of developing allyship.

WHAT LIES BENEATH

We all hold bias, and filter our experiences in order to self-define and stay safe. Bias shapes preference, for example, in our joining particular groups and networks with which we resonate. In its most extreme form, bias can lead to prejudice, hate crime and social violence. Identifying and understanding the lens through which we see ourselves and our world is central to making conscious our implicit biases. This is crucial in a field which constellates identity and challenges what is held up as typical or normative. When established ideas are questioned, either from inquiring curiosity or proximity to personal crisis, we re-evaluate their authenticity. This is an intellectual, visceral and personal growth process, as well as being a political act – disquieting, painful, rewarding (see also Campbell, Constantino and Simpson, 2019).

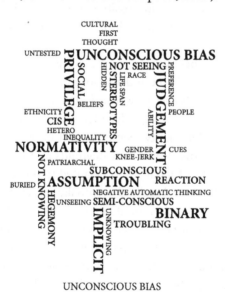

UNCONSCIOUS BIAS

CATCHING THE 'SECOND' THOUGHT

Initial negative automatic thoughts that chatter away in us tend to express a critical, biased commentary on ourselves and others. Noticing these, and reframing the subsequent, second thought enables a more processed, balanced perspective. In being interviewed for this book, Natasha shared the following reflection on how she came to acknowledge and work with her own implicit bias about her voice and vocal process.

Natasha (E, Psy): We all carry our own, often *unconscious biases* that affect the way we perceive the world. When I started re-training my voice (the first official training came at 18 months old, its second when testosterone hit me in puberty), I wanted to sound a lot more feminine. I wished for my voice to match my undeniably feminine presentation and appearance, and 'blend-in' as my gender – how I wanted others to see me. Putting all power onto how others perceive you can be terrifying; particularly because one can't actually control that. It's all so arbitrary and complex, dependent as much on internal and external environmental conditions (noise, lighting, moods, fatigue, emotionality) as on a billion other macro- and micro-factors. It's like trying to control the formation of waves in a vast ocean – wishing for all of them to roll a particular way.

What was seemingly impossible on the outside, became indeed possible for me. But I had to look elsewhere. I had to start *on the inside.*

My biggest block was not so much my ability to project a high pitched, 'sing-songy', soft and reassuringly timid feminine voice. It was my idea that *this* actually constituted feminine-sounding speak. Growing up with binary gender ideals, the apparent gap between masculinity and femininity seemed almost unbridgeable – especially in its 'purest' forms (think Burt Reynolds and Mariah Carrey). If I couldn't sound like Mariah, then I wanted to move as far away from Burt as possible. What I realized eventually was that pop culture, and more importantly my own socialization, was setting those benchmarks as they were. Socialization that occurred in a world dominated by gender inequality, like those paternalistic ideals often imposed on femininity; the prescriptive and often reductive formulas of female behavioural acceptability and respectability. A limited range, I found, and nowhere near as wide as the wonderful human vocal range we all possess!

In voice therapy, I came to realize that an open-minded, growing level of personal acceptance was equally important in training my voice so as to sound as I wanted. And that accepting *what is* with *no shame,* was key. When I let go of remorse for an undeniably difficult life thus far, overshadowed by a testosterone-infused puberty that permanently altered my vocal capacities, I am able to work with what I have. Work *with,* rather than against it, as friends or siblings. And help it/me explore and expand further. Instead of transforming my voice from a cube into a sphere, I slowly opened up to the idea of expanding the cube enough so as to fit the sphere inside (and pyramids too, if I ever so wanted!).

My single suggestion from experience, going out to all cis and gender-variant speech and language therapists/pathologists/voice specialists in trans voice, is to become friends with your unconscious biases. Bring them into the light of awareness and *gently* challenge them, moving from socialized limitations of norms and rigid gender stereotypes into the beautiful world of nuance. Avoiding this important introspection risks the work and output becoming one-dimensional, oddly mechanized and – regrettably – void of spirit.

My speech and language therapist was very aware of their internalized projections onto what constitutes these impossible to attain, yet heavily policed binary gender expectations. This facilitated a deeper exploration and awareness in me of my own unconscious biases regarding gender and voice. And consequently, I aimed to sound *proudly* like my feminine, complex self rather than a timid, copycat version of the wonderful Miss Carey.

Catching the second thought means, then, acknowledging those first judgmental thoughts arising in us, and softening them with awareness and compassion. Taking committed action with awareness means change is inevitable (Harris, 2007).

Daniella (E): At the end of the day, we are all human. We're all human – we have different experiences but we are all human. As I walk along my path of life, my history becomes my teacher.

PAUSE FOR REFLECTION:

- Recall the times when critical labels were applied to you, or when you may have reached for knee-jerk judgement of others.

- What were these labels?

- How might you reframe these thoughts with kindness?

IN THE FLASK: CISHETERONORMATIVITY

Cisheteronormativity is the status quo which views inhabiting and travelling through the world as cisgender (cis) and heterosexual as normal. It is not necessarily assumed that everyone in this system is cis and heterosexual, but if we are not, we are likely to be viewed as abnormal, even deviant. This is the social, political, legal and cultural construct of power and hierarchy in which we are all located and by which we are all affected. It is pervasive. It shapes our value systems and biases. Collectively, consciously or unconsciously, we contribute to codifying how privilege is stacked up and performed within normative rules and standards – who's in, who's not, what's in, what's not. We are locked in – analogous to the alchemist's hermetically sealed flask where the elements react and the drama initiates. Only when the new alchemical substance emerges, new awareness and perspective, can we break the seal and move the process on.

LPT (E): We are all constrained by a system which does not allow us to be whatever we want to be. I would say the cis hetero patriarchal normative system is a kind of prison in which we are all shackled and policed very violently.

And the thing is, no one can measure up to the cisnormative ideal in that system! Even that cis hetero white man bank manager is killing himself because he is not measuring up to his own construction of masculinity. Yeah, it's fucked. I would say that the speech and language therapist can't do this work unless they are psychologically aware of themselves and their own otherness in this system, so as not to dump shame onto their trans clients.

PAUSE FOR REFLECTION:

- Recall any time in your life when you felt you did not measure up to an expectation, when you felt you were not a fully accepted and paid up member to a significant group in your life.

- What contributed to you being treated as other or different? What thoughts and feelings arose in you? How did you cope?

Rachel (SLT): At the end of my first clinical placement day at the Gender Clinic, I felt like I had stepped through the looking glass. My eyes had been opened to a new sense of the world. I developed an acute awareness of cisnormative privilege and I connected with my own sense of being 'other' in my own life.

Normativity works to render non-normative identities and expressions invisible and non-existent. We concur with Beattie and Lenihan (2018) who argue that gender identity is universal. Cisheteronormative experience tends to 'locate challenges and skills in the *other*' (2018, p.16). However, gender identity is something we all have, perform and may explore, and happens not solely to a group of 'other people out there' whose gender identity may cause them issues for living.

Sean (SLT): The world as we have it will see *otherness* as problematic in some form or another. It's important to talk about being proud of who we are and what we have achieved in terms building our identities.

Privilege – conferring special rights and immunities – is often invisible to those who have it. Professor of Law, Alex Sharpe, activist, barrister and scholar in gender and sexuality, has challenged many 'gender identity fraud' prosecutions. In her EPATH 2018 keynote address she laid bare privilege as endowing the advantage of being able to look and choose not to see. A pedestrian, for example, who has already set off on a designated road crossing but is cut across by vehicle or cyclist, is rendered inferior and invisible in that moment. Whilst such an episode may seem trifling, it contains the subtle power-grab and micro- (perhaps macro-) aggression exerted by the advantaged road user who sees and chooses to ignore. 'To ensure real, progressive change, it is vital that those of us with any form of privilege use it to lift others up, rather than to simply pursue our own personal goals' (Pearce, 2018, p.17).

Anny (SLT): Being on placement at the Gender Identity Clinic has challenged my views on how I see the world. It's as though a filter has been removed and I can see a new spectrum of colour. I can now see how society moulds and moves us into people we think we've chosen to be. It's challenged my own identity and perception of self – how unconsciously I have contributed to 'norms' and biases and how I shall now, consciously, not do it. It's made me appreciate the beauty of self-expression and that we're all human beings who should be celebrated.

Developing consciousness of our environment, our *position* within it and how power structures work upon us, changes the inter- and intrapersonal landscape. The unconscious becomes conscious and the implicit, explicit (White, 2007). The Greek god of the underworld is Hades whose name means 'the unseen'. He is guardian of hidden treasure and symbolizes the bringing of new perspectives into conscious light. Hades allowed the buried treasure from the underworld to be revealed seasonally – symbolized by his wife Persephone who visits the earth in spring and represents the emergence of new life.

Christina (E): There isn't an average transgender person. I am Christina. There is a debate about trans women being in cis women's spaces. I think about labels – but for me – everyone is different. Some people do not want to be brought to thinking about their birth assigned gender, or to think about their chromosomes or biological history. Some trans people are okay with it. For me, go with what someone is saying right now. This is who I am, I don't speak for other trans people – I am not sure anyone can speak for other people – but we all have the right to our experience and that celebrates diversity. We're all human and it's a massive spectrum: some people are activist, some people want to blend into so-called normal (what is that, right?!) society as best as they can, some people want to reject it, some people are bold and open about being trans, others live in stealth and fear, there are many kinds of cis people, many kinds of trans people. The take home message is this: let people be individuals.

THE REAL DEAL?

It is necessary gently to examine our internalized cis-sexist perspective in our interactions. Do we have at the edges of our consciousness a view of our role as enabling the trans or non-binary person to be cis enough in order to thrive and survive? Are we sitting with the background thought: 'cis is the real deal; I am the real deal man/woman'? Many therapy approaches available in the market place are useful, yet the focus on enabling trans people to acquire 'passing privilege' is implicit.

LPT (E): Capitalism and commodification – the apps are making somebody money, but not the people who are using them.

Through dialogue and training with trans and non-binary people and groups, we can examine if we have subtly *othered* alternative versions of womanhood, manhood, in-between-hood queer identity in our thinking and behaviour (see Chapter 2). The antidote for everyone is to discover and look gently at privileges bestowed upon us.

LPT (E): Gender, class and race are the proverbial elephant in the room. From my experience and impression of the speech and language therapy profession, therapists seem predominantly middle class, probably white, mostly cis-het women. You know the archetypal 'nice white lady' who does good and means well. You know the ones who see themselves as politically liberal and open minded. Yet blindly unaware of their own race and class privilege.

If you are unconscious of your identity bias that is a barrier in itself to those trans people who are not cis, het or middle class. The white cis-het middle-class woman is coming with her whole history to the interaction, and people like me haven't been at the good end of that history. Black people or working-class people haven't had a good history of her type of woman. They need to know that they are coming in the room with baggage and look at their privilege.

I don't know the struggles of a cisgender woman in relation to voice and in relation to gender apart from certain beauty standards which deem certain bodies/voices undesirable and cisgender women feel the weight of that. This is different to what trans people experience. However, there are overlaps in trans people also being pressured to fulfil cisnormative beauty standards too. So how can we deconstruct our own understandings of gender in a safe way? Once you start to unravel that, it's going to have consequences for the rest of your life because there are a lot of ways in which you wanted to flex but felt that you just can't because of your husband or wife, children, etc. It's going to create a ripple effect once you start to question those things. But I think it is essential if you are a speech therapist or voice tutor in this field, you are going to have to question gender, and let it question you. You 'nice white lady' are going to have to question all your assumptions, for example, about black men.

Sean (SLT): My other clinical interest is bilingualism. People talk about cultural competence in bilingualism, quite rightly, because people have a different life from you – I would not expect my clients to have the same culture, religion, eating habits, etc.; people's perspective on the world is different. And that has an enormous impact if we don't take that into consideration. We can't work effectively with our clients, and the same is true with trans and non-binary clients. We're not the same. Even though I am gay, I am not the same as someone who is trans. All I can say is, I have some common ground and I would like to use that experience to show that you can work towards a sense of yourself which matters to you. If you are a cis, hetero, white female therapist as most SLTs are, it's not that you can't work with trans people – that's obviously nonsense, of course you can – but it's being mindful that your identity makes all sorts of assumptions about how people might be. For example, trans people are not some sort of 'lower class' of people. This idea that you have to feel sorry for people. Fortunately, that is probably less around now.

IT'S OKAY TO BE TRANS

It is highly relevant to know the history of pathologization of trans and non-binary people within medical care. Not so very long ago, and still present in some healthcare settings, being trans was conceptualized as a disorder to be fixed. This has been deeply harmful and damaging, the effects of which are still felt. Gender identity was set in binary cement, and the professional clinical group foregrounded its expertise over lived experience, and trans people have felt required to 'prove' their trans-ness with narratives that fit diagnostic descriptors in order to access desired services. It is beyond this book to examine the advantages and disadvantages of gate-keeping and informed consent models of service. Certainly, and absolutely, no medic, clinician and professional can diagnose a trans or non-binary identity (Vincent, 2018). Gladly, trans health care has stepped up to centring lived experience in affirmative ways, and trans is no longer seen as a disorder, though in a socialized healthcare system, diagnosis facilitates treatment funding (Richards *et al.*, 2015). Clinicians attempt to establish and understand the client's gender dysphoria, which is distress relating to their gender identity. See Vincent (2018) for a detailed account of the differences between diagnostic manuals in the field: the International Classification of Diseases of the World Health Organization, and the Diagnostic Statistical Manual of American Psychiatric Association.

Specialist centres, referred to as 'gender identity clinics' or 'gender dysphoria centres', aim to provide a supportive space for the trans and non-binary person to explore their gender identity, and offer triadic (bio-psycho-social) interventions which alleviate gender dysphoria in safe and sustainable ways (Barrett, 2017). Voice and communication therapy and exploration sits within the psychosocial trajectory. Gender specialist clinicians diagnose, risk assess and sign off on endocrine and surgical interventions – they 'ultimately decide if, when and how a transition should proceed' (Pearce, 2018, p.221). Due to pressures on services – workforce issues and lengthy waiting times – trans and non-binary people receive varied service provision in terms of geographic access and quality of care. The resilience, flexibility and creativity on the part of the trans and non-binary person needed to cope with waiting gives rise to what Pearce calls 'trans temporality' (2018, p.121). Developing networks, focus groups, clinical credentialing, competency frameworks, and accredited training and inclusive commissioning are beginning to tackle the crisis head on for the next generation (Mills *et al.*, 2018; Seal and Higgison, 2019). It is important to understand that many trans and non-binary people do not seek medical transition.

There are many compassionate multidisciplinary medics and non-medics who centre the trans person's expertise, and work creatively within the care system as it currently exists. We hope to foreground ways in which clients and clinicians can co-collaborate at the intersections of their experience. We acknowledge and emphasize that there is not a cis-clinician trans-client binary, and that trans and non-binary people may be both clinicians and clients.

Mary (SLT): I think the biggest thing, especially for a speech therapist who has been working with a different client populace, particularly in community or acute, is that idea of de-pathologization. Not treating trans-ness as a pathology. There may be a tendency for speech and language therapists to lean towards the medical aspects of 'treatment'. Even if you are a medical practitioner, the relationship approach shouldn't be one that centres on pathology or difference.

I think this applies to any populace that you work with in that you have a level of expertise about something, but, for example, if you are working with someone with aphasia, they have a level of expertise about the language they use, and how they want to be using language, and if you are working with someone who has a swallowing problem, they have expertise about their dietary habits, and whether or not they want to risk feed, etc. The person you work with has expertise about themselves and the world they live in. Often inadvertently, especially with really vulnerable people, there becomes a power dynamic, and I think trans is one populace where it can become really evident, because you are working with someone who is cognitively able and if the therapist is attached to the dynamic of 'I am the expert', it's completely the wrong approach to take. So, the approach has to be really one of acknowledging someone's expertise about their own voice, their own experience, and not making assumptions – not making assumptions about whether or not someone is misgendered, not making assumptions about whether or not someone wants a voice that 'passes' (if that's their language), or that being misgendered bothers someone. Leaving room for the scope of voices and acknowledging that it is an exploratory process, and that there is risk involved. The risk can be misgendering, it can be actual physical danger, but the most common way risk manifests is the conflict in where the person is now and where the person wants to be, and it can be traumatic, difficult to navigate – 'why is it so difficult for me to be myself?' or 'why is it so difficult to sound like myself?'

Jenny-Anne (E): I think it is important to receive some trans awareness training by trans people – it's really important to meet trans people, so a visit to the local support group or, as we did with our speech and language therapists in Cheshire where I was based, my therapist asked me to come and give a talk, and I know that you have done that in London at the Tavistock Clinic, and that of course Sean Pert has done this in Manchester too with his students.

We all learn from coming together. It's important to use literature and practice guides that have lived experience perspective embedded deeply within it as a collaborative enterprise. It reflects reality and honours the community. I think people can learn so much from visiting a local support group – all sorts of professionals come to visit our groups in Manchester, Cardiff and Llandudno, give a talk about what they do and come and chat to our members. What it does when anyone meets any minority is that it debunks the myths – so that people say, 'Oh, you are just ordinary people, and you are actually quite nice!' It's almost an insult, but we understand what people are saying and that people mean well [laughter].

PAUSE FOR REFLECTION:

- Trans singer-songwriter and activist, Justin Vivian Bond stated in an interview in *The Guardian* (Hoby, 2011): 'I think everybody's trans.'

- How does that resonate with you?

- Recommended reading: *Life Isn't Binary* (Barker and Iantaffi, 2019) and *Trans Like Me* (Lester, 2017).

KNOWLEDGE OF TERMS

Richards and Barker (2013, p.4) state:

> In the complex world of gender, sexuality and relationships, if one thing is assured it is that you will inadvertently offend someone, not uncommonly a group of people you were previously unaware of. Kindness and continuing education are key. This involves having good intentions and being mindful of the impact even well-intended words and behaviours actually have.

We offer some suggested terminology as a practical overview supported by lived experience.

Skye (E, Psy): It's gender so it's messy! I see trans as an umbrella term referring to people who don't identify with the gender they were assigned at birth, which would include non-binary people. We say trans and non-binary because there are some non-binary people who don't use the label trans. For a while I was reluctant to use that label myself when I first identified as non-binary. Our idea of what it is to be trans(gender) is very binary, and some non-binary people may feel that they are encroaching on a space that isn't theirs.

Terminology is rapidly evolving. People new to the field can feel a great deal of anxiety initially because they do not want to 'get it wrong', slip up, appear gauche, rude or say something offensive. Trying to hold an encyclopaedic knowledge through rote-learning terms, though, produces further anxiety and fixedness. It is important to understand the epistemological underpinnings and history of terms, but affirmative practice is most importantly and essentially about checking out with people. We refer you to Pearce (2018), Vincent (2018), Barker and Iantaffi (2019), Lester (2017) and Iantaffi and Barker (2018) for deeper discussion of terms. Respectfully adopting the 'ask etiquette' (Richards and Barker, 2015, p.39) with the trans and non-binary person who has come to consult with you is recommended by experts by experience. 'When in doubt, ask' (Vincent, 2018, p.20).

The most fundamental point is that everyone's gender identity is a unique and personal experience. It is not up for grabs by anyone but ourselves, though we may seek help to explore its expression and how we negotiate ourselves in social, including cyber, context over time.

Transgender (synonymous with 'trans' derived from the Latin meaning 'across from') describes an individual whose gender identity does not match their gender assigned at birth. Note that if an individual identifies as a trans man or a trans woman, the 'trans' is adjectival and separate, and used only when pertinent and with the individual's consent. We are in no way suggesting that the trans identity is to be hidden, spoken about *sotto voce* or cast quickly into the shadows, to coin Christine Burns' phrase (2019), but the disclosure story rests wholly with the trans person. 'Transfeminine' and 'transmasculine' are adjectives meaning 'more feminine' and 'more masculine', respectively and may be used by non-binary and binary trans people.

Cisgender (usually contracted to 'cis', deriving from the Latin prefix meaning 'on this side of') describes an individual whose gender identity matches their gender assigned at birth.

Non-binary describes an individual whose gender identity transcends the male and female dichotomy. As with trans, non-binary is an overarching term describing many experiences of further genders, where individuals have a gender identity that is androgynous, neutral, neither exclusively male or female, between male and female, fluid and variable over time, bi-gender, multiple genders, or agender. Genderqueer is largely synonymous with non-binary, but has historically evoked more political connotations in its rejection of typical and fixed notions of gender roles and performance (Barker and Iantaffi, 2019; Richards, Bouman and Barker, 2017; Vincent, 2018).

Pearce (2018) and Vincent (2018) identify shadow terms, which may be less favoured, obsolete or cause offence. These may include: Male-to-Female (MtF), Female-to-Male (FtM), transgenders (used as a noun), sex change, born male/female, transpeople/transwoman/transman (used as a single noun and implying that someone's entire identity is predicated on being trans), passing. The corollary of identifying safe or 'safer terms' (Richards and Barker, 2013, p.4) is that the 'wrong' terminology is unsafe and dangerous, leading to fear of saying the wrong thing and walking on egg shells. Indeed, clinicians and practitioners need to understand nuance, and most importantly, give space for trans and non-binary people to use those descriptors which are valid for them. This will foster respectful and collaborative interaction, so that the trans or non-binary person is asked what is best for them without being required to educate the clinician in detail about being trans.

INTERSECTIONALITY

Audre Lorde was a profound intersectional thinker and leader: 'there is no such thing as a single-issue struggle because we do not live single-issue lives' (1984/2019, p.133). First propounded by Black legal scholar Crenshaw (1989), intersectionality is a model which uncovers how systems of privilege and power interweave and interlock. It helps us understand how we are located on a privilege-oppression continuum. More, it enables us to make visible diversity and complexity where we have reached for cultural binary assumptions such as black-white, trans-cis, male-female, fluent-dysfluent, disabled-non-disabled, gay-straight, old-young, fat-thin, quick-slow, high-low (Barker and Iantaffi, 2019). When we begin to think intersectionally, we step away from centering patriarchal versions of events and people and allow people to reveal their own identity descriptors, meaning-making and privilege-oppression map (see figure: 'Intersectionality').

LPT (E): We are taught that gender is somehow separate from race, somehow separate from sexuality. And it's all connected. It's essential for speech therapists to understand, or have some training in intersectionality. And to centre people who are disenfranchised, which means trans women, who are black, working class, etc. Once you have that analysis in your head, everything falls better in place. You are not centring 'white male' as the norm. That surely will have relevance for how you account for, describe and measure or perceive voice. A black trans woman coming into a space is not going to be the same as a white trans woman. A trans woman of colour will come with a whole set of baggage and fear because, quite frankly, they are the most likely to be killed, of all of us trans people. So, it's important even to have the knowledge of the world of the people who you are dealing with.

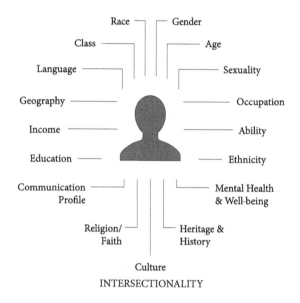

INTERSECTIONALITY

Pertinent to this, in a TEDx talk Ashlee Marie Preston speaks of her daily struggle and negotiation of transmysogynoir (the oppression of trans women and transfeminine people of colour): the intersection of transphobia, misogyny and anti-blackness (Preston, 2018).

QUEER

This a broad but very pertinent category included in the LGBTQIA+ acronym (lesbian, gay, bisexual, transgender, queer, intersex, aromantic/asexual/agender, and more) – see Barker and Scheele (2016). It originally meant 'strange'. We define queerness as a worm hole through the structure and temporality of cisheteronormativity, creating and expressing its own framework, qualitatively independent of any normative system and categorization. It rejects, challenges, is vocal and visible, and stands politically proud. It *gives the finger*.

Skye (E, Psy): Being queer and identifying as queer is an opposition to structure and categories which I think is very useful.

Mary (SLT): Queer is complex. There are so many different meanings of that, and there is an ongoing dialogue about who has the right to use that word because of its etymology as a slur. I'm someone who identifies as queer with a very specific meaning about my relationship to my sexuality, not as much my relationship to gender. It can become an umbrella for 'otherness'. My sense is that the risk with that umbrella is that there are queer spaces built by queer people for the safety of queer people – people whose lives are materially and legislatively affected by the facts of their gender or sexuality – that does not apply to everyone – and that queerness refers to a reclamation of that otherness and owning it for the purposes of advocating for that legislative and material protective advancement. But the way that people who are oppressed navigate the world and advocate for themselves is ultimately something that will liberate everyone. So, to connect this to voice: when we talk about queering the larynx, which is language that comes from the goals of one of our non-binary patients (I love that so much), I would interpret that as a deviating from the expectations that someone might have for someone's voice in relation to their gender, or not, or having the freedom to take on characteristics of the voice that is associated with gender while reclaiming and owning stereotypical aspects of it.

Queer is an umbrella term to express nonconformity in established gender and sexual identity. It champions ambiguity, questioning, independence and political action. Sylvia Rivera, veteran of the 1969 Stonewall uprising, famously declared: 'hell hath no fury like a drag queen scorned'.

COMING OUT

Coming out – the process of being open publicly or to a particular group about gender or sexuality – is costly because, in most cases, it means relating fundamentally to a shamed sense of self (there is more on this in Chapter 2). Whilst it can be liberating, it requires being ready and resilient enough to risk ridicule, rejection, violence, loss of family, friends, support, respect, income and home. It is never a single event and extends over one's life. Coming out as lesbian, gay or bisexual tends to be, but is not always, an invisible process to all but the subject until spoken out and named. That is not the case, generally, with coming out as trans, where physical, behavioural, vocal and social role changes are in the public domain, and loved ones, supporters, colleagues and strangers feel, often with good intention, that they can partake in them and comment on the trans or non-binary person's process, unsolicited. Every coming out experience is unique.

LPT (E): We can't pretend there are no costs for coming out. You can't come out, for example, in some industries because you will earn less money, or lose your job. Coming out as trans or LGB can very damaging. That's not to say you can't feel liberated at some level. Straight people don't come out. They never say 'I am straight. Hey I am straight!' Cis people never come out and say 'I am cis' unless they have made a conscious effort to do so. It's not needed, apparently, in the construct in which we live. It's *assumed*.

So, people who are not trans or LGBT can fill in forms without thinking 'oh where is my gender'. It's not cis or straight people's fault. It's systemic. But when you wake up to realizing you don't match up and you have to *come out*, it's a really tough process. And even though there is more legislature around to protect minorities, there's a rise in xenophobia, transphobia, racism etc. and some people act on feelings of hate violently. That's the extreme, but we are all in it together. Speech therapists – please know that you can make a difference by making conscious your own bias. Don't give a politically correct, lip-service therapeutic practice. Bring yourself to genuinely embrace difference and know the lens you are looking through is biased. It's the only way forward in offering a transformative process for your clients.

Remember ticking 'straight' on a form can be done by people who identify as straight, without thinking there may be a cost, at the declaration of your sexual orientation. But we don't know how this information/data is going to be used in the future. We do not have to be paranoid to understand that we live in a world where often our personal data is harvested and used without our permission in many instances. In addition, the neural pathways for non–LGBTQ+ folk are likely not geared for 'alert, alert, alarm, alarm!' in the disclosure of being cis or straight, in the way that if you are trans or LGBTQ+, we do have those little triggers – what does this mean? For what purposes am I being recorded? Can I trust someone in my absence to tell my story honestly, and not spin it to their own professional or financial ends?

There is a deeper positive to be gained, though. For me personally, I see I can attract different kinds of people into my life that are more real, that can be more real with me because I am being more real generally and to myself. We probably won't be able to say though 'I am cured of heteropatriarchy. Jesus!! Thank you! Hallelujah!'

Sean (SLT): It's over 50 years since Stonewall. It was trans women who did most of the work for that because they were so far away from society's idea of the norm, whatever that is. It's a cultural competence to understand this history because it informs the life experience of most people who are queer in some regard or another. We don't just come out once – we come out constantly. I was working with a trans woman who had what might be typically understood as such a feminine gender expression, including voice, that she would never be misgendered or seen as anything other than normatively female/feminine, and she came as a volunteer, and I was wearing a 'some people are trans, get over it!' t-shirt and she said to me, 'I couldn't wear that t-shirt.' And I asked why, and she said, 'It's my worst nightmare for people to know that I am trans.' And I said, 'I think you still have some work to do, which is why you probably volunteered. Being proud of being trans is something to aim for.' And she did end up hanging out with a group on Canal Street and feeling far more connected to her identity.

THE COST OF AUTHENTICITY

Exploring, creating and sustaining voice and communication, as we have written, centres client flexibility and self-concept at the core. Supporting clients through the processes of 'start smart', 'press on' and 'finish strong' (Hancock and Siegfriedt, 2020) and enabling them to code switch authentic voice in situational context is a journey of obstacles, challenges and victories. LPT attended one of our transmasculine voice groups, and describes their experience.

LPT (E): In the transmasculine voice group we talked about the cost of authenticity. There's always a cost. We wear series of masks as we negotiate day-to-day activities in the world. It's like we have one persona at work, another at home, another on the street, depending on how safe we feel, and the challenge always is to integrate as a whole and not wear a mask. But I don't know whether that is possible in the world. I genuinely don't know. Often there's a conversation amongst, for example, black people about code switching so there are ways that you are in white context and ways that you behave that are very different in black context. The white context is often about employment and survival, so people choose ways that are about survival which might not be good for mental health, but they get you paid. Do you see what I am saying?

And so, to be your authentic self, could possibly lose you your job. Particularly if you are of colour, particularly if you are gender nonconforming. A lot of being your authentic nonconforming gendered way might lead you to your death. Do you see? So, there is a cost, a dangerous, maybe deadly, cost to be truly authentic. But at the same time it might be your salvation.

This is experience richly described and the learning is sobering. It teaches the importance of understanding both potential benefits and risks to being authentic. Authenticity is perilous and cannot be a term used glibly. Preparing for realistic expectation and the possibility of difficult times ahead, developing flexibility, code-switching, resilience, self-efficacy and community support – are factors to mitigate risk (see Chapters 2 and 4).

SAFE SPACE?

Further to the cost of authenticity, we wish to touch on the troubling socio-political debate about trans women in women's safe spaces. Patel (2017) writes about violent 'cistems' and trans experience of bathroom or toilet space. Nirta (2018) discusses marginalization of trans bodies. This is the view that trans women are considered to have or retain male privilege and take up or claim a 'masculine' amount of space and time.

Skye (E, Psy): Some say that trans women take up more space than cis women, and would use this to argue against the inclusion of trans women in women's spaces. One of the assumptions underlying this idea is that trans women have male privilege. However, I think it's worth noting that AMAB [assigned male at birth] and AFAB [assigned female at birth] people are all taught the same gender power dynamic (i.e. patriarchy) which gets internalized by everyone. How you relate to that power dynamic can be influenced by your presentation and how you are treated by others, but also by your own internal sense of gender identity. Trans women can still internalize the same ideas about femininity that cis women do (e.g. that you shouldn't take up space, that you should be quiet, that you should be deferential) even before they start expressing their gender identity. So, I don't think it's so straightforward that an AMAB person goes through their life with male privilege even if they are presenting as a man.

It's also important to remember that, statistically, trans women are at higher risk of abuse, sexual harassment, domestic violence and murder than cis women. So, if it's a case of protecting people who are vulnerable, trans women have just as much a right to be in those safe spaces as cis women.

Marginalized groups of any kind may express protest and reclaim power by tightly defining the inclusion criteria for membership of the group, and may push into the unconscious what socio-political privilege, however nuanced, it may be endowed with. This leads to a cycle of intersectional oppression – cis women who marginalize trans women and straight men who marginalize gay men are just two examples.

PAUSE FOR REFLECTION:

- What is your position on the debate about socialized privilege?
- Reflect on normative perceptions of size of bodies, size of voice and the stereotypes these may attract in our understanding of so-called gender spaces.

CN Lester, academic, writer, classical mezzo-soprano and co-founder of the UK's first national queer youth organization, speaks eloquently of *inclusive feminism* as something we do rather than something we are. Transphobic feminism is a minority, often expressed by trans-exclusionary radical feminists (TERFs) (Smythe, 2018) and tends towards narrow definition and closed membership. When feminism occupies a generous space, it becomes a toolbox that everyone can contribute to and share in (Lester, 2018).

Stephen (E, M): I think a lot of trans people are anxious about being put into a box. When we go for medical treatment, there is quite a strong pull of 'you are jumping from column A to column B' as it were, and proving that you belong in that new column. Maybe more so historically than now, but this view persists. And there is a lot of fear around that because there is a feeling that you will have to prove yourself or you may be denied care, so I think particularly if people have come through the NHS or socialized medicine, there's probably some fear about whether they measure up to that category and/or being put in that category when maybe they are non-binary, but saying 'the correct' thing in order to qualify for what they want out of the system, which I think happens a lot. This translates vocally as: it is important to explore your voice and vocal technique, rather than trying to 'masculinize' or 'feminize' your voice, because that feels like it's a pass-fail. Ideas of 'fully feminizing voice' are kind of horrific (and I have heard those judgements come from clinical viewpoints) and are to be avoided.

OUR PRACTICE: USING INCLUSIVE LANGUAGE

We have already considered that it is understandable for developing professionals to worry about using so-called outmoded terms, and that the remedy is always to ask politely of our clients. Misgendering (using pronouns, descriptors or 'deadnames' [Vincent, 2018, p.24] which contradict someone's identity) manifests from the assumption that cis is ubiquitous, or comes from a momentary slip up and lack of specificity. It is affirmative for cis people to own their cisness and pronouns *in the first instance* entirely matter-of-factly, thereby normalizing the practice without othering or pressurizing the trans person.

LPT (E): I'd say therapists start with themselves first, and say, '*My* gender pronouns are whatever, whatever, whatever. What gender pronouns do you use?' I think always start from the *I*, because if you start from the other person, it's saying they are *othered*. From my understanding, the majority of speech and language therapists are cis, and if they seem to be welcoming and then ask the trans or gender nonconforming person their gender pronouns first, it others the trans person. So, better to say, 'Mine are these, what are yours?' Just as *you* did actually.

Skye (E, Psy): I would say the positive thing is that being an ally is not complicated. The solution is quite straightforward – people who want to be allies should speak with trans people and ask them what language they would like you to use, what services they want to access and how they might best support them.

Jenny-Anne (E): I like to say that we are both different and the same. Isn't that true of all human beings? Then there's not a discord. My feeling is that, if for whatever reason, you have never had to interact with a minority, you have never had to investigate or learn about it, why should you know? Although some people may not agree with that. People don't know because they don't know and often, though not always, people don't engage in an attempt not to offend, people are afraid of getting it wrong. And then the community thinks they are being stand-offish and critical.

Misgendering? Just apologize and move on. Accept that you are wrong, move on. Don't make a big thing about it. Most people who are gender diverse know the difference between someone making a genuine slip or mistake, and someone being deliberately discriminatory or obnoxious. Most of the time, people simply get it wrong, because they have reacted subconsciously, with an established assumption and missed or not responded to the person's gender clues.

People in the trans community are also capable of making similar mistakes because gender is such a huge spectrum we can often get it wrong.

Someone who came to me for some advice was presenting in an extremely successful way in terms of typically perceived femininity, and I made the assumption when they said they were starting hormones that they were wishing to masculinize and start testosterone; actually, they were trans female and had just started oestrogen and I made the error of not checking with them to start with. I am human! Good to remember we all are. We all make assumptions, often subconsciously.

Using the 'epicene they' (Vincent, 2018, p.67) in referring to non-binary identifying people in the third person takes linguistic adjustment.

Practically, this means slowing down our talk and preparing ahead cognitively to make space for the appropriate language, especially in group conversations and when there is a time pressure. In the event that we do misgender someone, the community wisdom is to not burden the trans or non-binary person with over-apology, which has the effect of asking them to make it better for you. Apologize succinctly and move on.

Skye (E, Psy): Worrying about getting things wrong is an understandable feeling for people who want to be allies, but sometimes it can go too far the other way where someone is so worried about getting something wrong that they centre their own role as an ally, rather than considering the feelings of the trans person. So, if you misgender someone it's much better to apologize and move on rather than make a big deal about it.

For a lot of people, gender neutral pronouns might be a new thing, or using new pronouns for someone might take some time to get used to. I think trans people are generally sympathetic to that. If someone makes a mistake, it's important that they don't then make the situation about them and their status as an ally, but to move on. Otherwise the trans person may feel the need to console the person who misgendered them – telling them 'it's okay...' and that becomes extra emotional labour for them.

Referring to someone's assigned gender at birth is also best avoided, though in the context of some interventions (notably surgical) it may be a short-hand for some clinicians. We say more about 'de-gendering the larynx', particularly in respect of working with non-binary people, in Chapter 3.

Skye (E, Psy): Where possible, I would avoid foregrounding the gender someone was assigned at birth which, for many trans people, is not something they want to focus on. There are ways for the clinician and patient to discuss the voice without having to refer to birth assignation.

Using inclusive language also means re-examining the nomenclature of our interventions (see Chapter 3). We recommend readers access the YouTube channel 'ContraPoints' run by Natalie Wynn (2019), trans activist and cultural commentator, who provides a searingly witty and critical commentary on being trans in a complex world.

Mary (SLT): ContraPoints made a post that said she really hated when she is in a group of cis people and someone decides that we need to do a pronoun-around – it makes her feel that she has been clocked, outed. Although it benefits some trans people, for her, it actually induces dysphoria, and she said that we should think how this affects trans people who pass. Many non-binary people were up in arms about this – pronoun-around benefits people who don't use binary pronouns! In our groups, if we ask people to share their pronouns, people are often really not interested, they just want people to assume their pronouns. Passing privilege is the ability to mitigate risk by being stealth or having choice in when and where you reveal your trans-ness. Important to note that a cis person cannot ascribe 'passing privilege' to a trans person. One of our psychiatrists tells patients to go for strong cues about your gender expression – people will know what you are doing and they will be less confused, and people will leave you alone. I am not sure that is true, but there is something for non-binary people being in a space where people can't tell what your gender is – this is optimal for them and gender affirming, but actually in many ways leads them to a sense of risk because often confusion provokes anger for people if they don't know what gender someone is. So, there is a level of visibility and vulnerability for non-binary people that some more binary trans people don't have.

Skye (E, Psy): 'Feminization' and 'masculinization' are very broad labels, but there is some common understanding about what they mean in our culture, and I think there will be lots of trans people who are totally fine with using these terms. It's just a matter of the therapist asking the service user how they would like to talk about their voice. Some clients won't have the specific language or concept understanding to name component vocal parts very specifically in the early stages of therapy and may rely on generalized gendered concepts. But the more you steer people towards what specific changes they want, rather than relying on normative ideas of what it is to have a 'masculine' or 'feminine' voice, the better I think. You can still explore the parameters of voice without getting too jargon-orientated.

It is not for the professional to judge or dissuade a client from a binary construction of self and the world. It is okay to identify as binary trans and binary cis. Moreover, affirming an 'and, and' perspective in the consultation is more helpful than a reductive 'either, or' perspective, and enables flexibility in choice that may not have been previously known. In a time where rigid binary thinking which protects privilege and propagates oppositional conflict, wreaking havoc globally on our political and eco systems, flexibility and creativity are desperately needed (Barker and Iantaffi, 2019; Lester, 2017).

BEING A TRANS ALLY: BEYOND THE THERAPY ROOM

Audre Lorde pointed the way: 'without community, there is no liberation...but community must not mean a shedding of our differences, nor the pathetic pretense that these differences do not exist' (1984/2019, p.105). Once we know what we know, we cannot un-know it. We have a social and civil responsibility to speak up when we judge a situation to be harmful to others. Ashlee Marie Preston states that 'acknowledgement without action is aid and abetment' (2018).

Skye (E, Psy): If someone works with trans people, or any another minority group, and never interacts with those people outside of work, I think it's important to reflect on why that might be and how that might influence how they see their patients.

The topic of gender identity at the moment is so politicized. I don't expect clinicians to start marching in the street, but I think it is important to see trans people as part of a community in its political context not just as individual patients who are just part of your job.

Mary (SLT): Make trans friends. Know that you have trans family (the chances are there are people that are related to you or in your proximity that are trans whether or not you know it). Honestly, advocate politically for trans people because there's no use doing this work if the world isn't safe for people to be themselves in. It's completely pointless for people to come in to your clinic room and do an hour or so work with them and then they have to go back out into a world where they could be murdered. You have to be a compassionate person to do this job well, and I think to be an actually compassionate person, you have to believe in their well-being – materially, legislatively, and in terms of safety (protective factors), in the ability for people to live a life that is as good as you live. You have to believe those things in order to do this job well. In order to work compassionately in a field, your compassion has to extend as far as really believing that everyone else deserves the kind of life that you have, that everyone has access to the things you have – that's not just for trans people.

We're just a part of enabling trans people to live as people. Some people will have trans-ness at the forefront of their identity because it's a choice they want to make, some people just want to get on with their lives and not have you see them as a trans person first.

Cis people can help to normalize social add-ons that trans people may need to do in the workplace. Stating our pronouns in conversation, at the beginnings of meetings and including them in email signatures means these practices become matter-of-fact. If someone misgenders an absent trans friend or colleague, correct them and move on.

We all have a responsibility to challenge top-down thinking which structurally excludes trans and non-binary people, queer-identifying people and people expressing themselves beyond normative expectation. Celebrating diversity becomes active when we are able to discuss our work openly, and gently challenge assumption and ignorance in our families, friendships and in the workplace. In this way, we dissolve pity, voyeuristic, blameful and rescue narratives.

Skye (E, Psy): Include trans people as much as possible in research, decision-making and policy. Like this book. You are valuing the lived and unique experiences of trans people. For so long, things have been divisive between the trans community and the clinical professionals who work with them. We have a lot of work to do to close that gap. It's not enough to pay lip service to that dialogue, we should consult with the community when making decisions. Trans people are the experts of their own lived experience.

No more top down decisions without any community engagement.

LPT (E): The speech therapist can't say 'I am a trans ally now' and go out into the world and not challenge anything. That's nonsense, because you will bring that energy or way of interacting back into the therapy with you. It won't do. If being a trans ally is just within the four walls of the clinic, it's not going to work, you are not going to have that sort of fluid energy of 'I am really part of the changing dialogue, I am really actively part of it'. You have to be. You can't just switch on and off your trans ally status. It's not really good enough and it requires a little bit more work – I mean that in a gentle but challenging way. Because you are vocal alchemists, vocal psychotherapists, and you are dealing with people's lives and their vulnerabilities, that can cut them to the core. Voice is about identity, at the core.

Naz (SLT): It's all about being reflexive. It's important for speech and language therapists, sole practitioners or those who work at arm's length from other specialists, actively to make links and stay connected to the voice community. If we stay in silos and don't have an ongoing dialogue, whatever level or experience we are working at, we risk becoming complacent, out of date or stuck in our ways. We need dialogue so colleagues can pick up on things, ask your rationale, check your competence, including cultural competence, and important for us to have someone to think aloud with. It's desperately important to have that time and space to reflect in supervision – but the supervisee sets the agenda. The supervisor is not an examiner, or an oracle, or there to 'tell you' information, but there as a guide who can help you dig a bit deeper into the question and reflection. So, it's important, for SLTs working far from others or as sole practitioners to reach out: your supervisor, we hope, will be a skilled clinician also in the process.

I think of myself as a speech therapist first, a voice therapist as the next tier, then as a gender specialist trans voice and communication therapist as the next tier up, but keeping abreast of what's going on culturally, vocally and psychologically. The North-East Voice CEN gives me opportunities to see who else is working with trans clients (people I work with at the Newcastle Gender dysphoria service) and we have a robust network of sharing. I know this happens in other parts of the UK – the Scottish therapists are very organized in their networks, there's great work being done in the South West of England, and vibrant pockets – Manchester, Birmingham, Yorkshire, etc. Really important having and being part of our National CEN through the Royal College for support and networking, and British Association of Gender Identity Specialists (BAGIS) for multi-professional learning

Again, we champion Lorde: 'we have to consciously study how to be tender with each other until it becomes a habit' (1984/2019, p.171).

Reflexivity facilitates freedom, flexibility and an ability to respond, rather than react, with thought and compassionate action. We become responsible, affirmatively response-able.

SUMMARY:

- Make your unconscious bias conscious, towards a compassionate, thought-out positionality.

- Own your own slice of privilege.

- Come out as cis and state your pronouns first, rather than othering the trans person.

- Know the legislature, respect confidentiality and do not out the trans person.

- Use affirmative terms and adopt an ask etiquette approach.

- Use inclusive language, describing individuals in the way they request.

- Apologize and move on in the event of misgendering.

- Meet the trans person where they are at in terms of who they are and what they want to work on.

- Respect the integrity and context of trans stories.

- Shift from using pity narratives and being a cis rescuer of trans people.

- Avoid expecting the trans person to be your trans educator.

- Avoid asking questions to satisfy your own curiosity about the process.

- Be a proud trans ally and speak about your work in many contexts.

CHAPTER 2

The Psychological Space

THERAPEUTIC ALLIANCE

THIS CHAPTER WILL ASK

What is psychological contact and how do we use approaches to co-create and maintain a therapeutic and practice space that supports the change process?

How do we build trust and acknowledge the paradox of change?

This chapter, as the first, is about relationship – relating to self, clients and the world in trans affirmative ways. The importance of the therapeutic relationship within the biopsychosocial model and the psychological approaches used to support client goals within voice and communication is well established (Adler, Hirsch and Pickering, 2019; Baker, 2017; Butcher, Elias and Cavalli, 2007; Caughter and Crofts, 2018; Cheasman, Everard and Simpson, 2013; DiLollo and Favreau, 2010; Flasher and Fogle, 2012; Fourie, 2009; Harley, 2015, 2018; James and Brumfitt, 2018; Kelman and Wheeler, 2015; Logan, 2013; Mills and Stoneham, 2017). Continuing professional development within counselling and psychotherapy will be determined by individual preferences and opportunities, and we have included only a few approaches here to stimulate reflection and illustrate practice.

PSYCHOLOGICAL CONTACT

We know fundamentally that in a therapy space, all that is in us is 'in the room' and all that is in the client is 'in the room'. This is what

Carl Rogers, pioneer of the person-centred approach, means by 'psychological contact' (1956/2004) and it is revealed though proximity, response and relationship. We review this therapeutic alliance and its relevance to trans affirmative practice: what do we set up spatially and contextually, and how does our social, clinical and therapeutic privilege intersect with the client's expertise and world view? It is helpful indeed if we have experienced and been 'held' in a therapy process of our own.

Having examined the view seen through the lens of cishetero-normativity, we have fertile ground to deal with greater complexity in clinical practice. This is achieved in the first instance by acknowledging that gender is a universal experience in which we are all positioned: 'even when gender is not the "problem", it is present and affecting process, transference and countertransference, and our ability to be fully present and empathic with our clients' (Beattie and Lenihan, 2018, p.15).

In essence, we can do no better than meet people where they are in themselves, and ask very simply 'how can I help you?' We are able then to take that first step with our client, an act of trust, and to ready for expedition to the unknown terrain. From this stance, everything else can follow well. We are enabling people *to be* and *to learn*; we too are in a being and learning process, which can be both shared and in parallel with our clients. It is all right not to know and feel like an imposter for both therapist and client. This is the most authentic place of psychological contact as it centers human-to-human meeting and being on the 'same page'. The 'therapeutic pyramid' proposed by Fife *et al.* (2014) usefully reminds us that we begin with a way of being, develop therapeutic alliance followed by a skills-based focus. Within the consultation, we front our expertise in voice at the same time as welcoming client expertise in their voice and their life. In our practice, we have found, in particular, Solution Focused Brief Therapy (De Shazer *et al.*, 2012), Narrative Therapy (White, 2007), mindfulness, (Kabat-Zinn, 1990, 2016; Segal, Williams and Teasdale, 2018) Compassion Focused Therapy (Gilbert, 2015) and image work (Malchiodi, 2012, 2018) are approaches which dovetail well with trans voice and communication, and are deeply helpful in facilitating enquiry beyond technique. We offer discussion of these through case study, client work and interviews with trans and non-binary people and specialist colleagues. These approaches are not presented as exhaustive or prescriptive.

WHO DO WE THINK WE ARE?

Let us start by asking ourselves the who, what, why questions of how we see our role.

PAUSE FOR REFLECTION:

- Which words best describe the way you see your role in the clinical and practitioner space?

- What professional badge(s) are you wearing when you come to trans and non-binary voice and communication work?

Do we foreground assessing, diagnosing, treating, planning, risk assessing, problem-solving and advising? *Naming* is a fundamental human process in manifesting identity and can prescribe and direct behaviour and attitude, including professional ways of being and doing (James and Brumfitt, 2018).

Annie (V): If you are in the room as a researcher you need to know that. Therapists give of themselves. 'I gave this advice then I went home at five o'clock.' No. Therapy of all kinds, including speech and language therapy, is a very deep enterprise and it doesn't stop at five o'clock or any o'clock – we have taken clients in and they have taken us in. Of course, we have professional boundaries, but clients may be traumatized, shamed, distressed, grieving, and we are carrying them over the distance and working towards our redundancy as they become skilled and self-efficacious. We are helping people to become whole.

Naz (SLT): I notice in my clinical work that the relevance for collecting objective data falls away. I have had people in their individual or final review, and I ask about their voice – how it is, what's working for them, how it is now. Rather than collecting a complete data set for me as a therapist to prove my worth, I ask if it would be meaningful to repeat an objective measure, and sometimes people say 'yes', and often people say 'no I don't think it will add anything to where I am now'. I end up with incomplete data sets, if you like, but relevant impact statements and meaningful therapeutic relationship.

THE DRAMA TRIANGLE

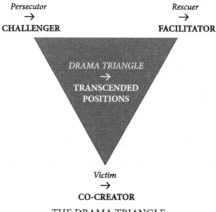

THE DRAMA TRIANGLE

Developed by Stephen Karpman (1968), a student of Eric Berne (1964/2010) who pioneered Transactional Analysis, the Drama Triangle offers a helpful model which we can use to better understand our role as therapist and practitioner, the power dynamics within the therapeutic relationship, and how expertise is negotiated and shared. In essence, it describes human dysfunctional relationships and social 'games' entered into by two or more individuals – the unconscious aim being to seek out and receive negative, in the absence of receiving positive, recognition. These are universal coping strategies developed in childhood which we default to in times of stress, anxiety and trauma. Three roles triangulate, with two 'up' (empowered) and one 'down' (disempowered) positions. We shift from one to another in quick succession, but the ultimate outcome is victimhood for all. They have the following broad characteristics (see Karpman, 2014):

- **Persecutor** – expresses frustration, self-righteousness, blame, aggressive or passive-aggressive behaviours. Narratives tend towards: 'I am right – you are in the wrong.'

- **Rescuer** – expresses sensitivity and often takes responsibility for other people's problems and makes them their own, rather than looking at their own life. Narratives tend towards saving and being parental: 'I am nice, I can help people, if they do what I say they will succeed and be happy.' There is a preference for fixing over discovering solutions inherent in the one being helped.

- **Victim** – expresses helplessness and feeling powerless. Narratives tend to disablement and injustice: 'I can't', 'it's not fair', 'rescue me'. There tends to be a lack of agency and self-worth, and of the confidence to be self-reliant.

We initiate interactions from a favoured 'starting gate' position, the role we see and prefer as (part of) our identity.

PAUSE FOR REFLECTION:

- What is your starting gate position?

- Do you have another preferred position, and one you tend to avoid?

The cycle is broken and we transform the three roles only by becoming increasingly conscious of what we are being invited and drawn into, and into what we invite and draw others. We likely become therapists because forming a helping relationship and validating people is important to who we are. In the therapy context, and in particular within a medical setting, though, we may unconsciously be drawn to the rescuer position, which places the clients at the centre of the healing process but may encourage dependency on clinical expertise over client self-efficacy. It can feel very facilitative, even satisfying, because we are responding to the client's unconscious desire to be rescued and returned to comfort and function. We have entered into that pact because clients arrive in states of distress, but what the client is actually doing is rescuing the therapist by enabling the therapist to feel potent and authoritative. These are some ways in which drama triangle positions exert influence, shift and oscillate rapidly. Similarly, in the context of assessing and diagnosing, where clinical expertise and authority is foregrounded, we may unconsciously be drawn to aspects of the persecutor. It is important to stress that these are largely *unconscious* processes, and extremely subtle. They link with personal psychological phenomena, how we align with and construct our professional identity, and how we discharge our responsibilities.

Annie (V): Unless we as therapists truly sacrifice those unconscious needs and actually risk being found out, being seen through, then we maintain the expert role and those secondary gains of being seen as *the expert.*

Over-identifying with clinical authority may mean we deny some of our vulnerability. We explore this in particular in Chapter 3 related to relational voice work. Intrinsic to working professionally, evidentially and confidentially, and to setting safe boundaries, it is appropriate in the first instance for therapists to accept and embody the archetype of expert from the client. The skill is then to hand the archetype of expert back gently and mindfully to the client by acknowledging and empowering their expertise in the course of therapy and exploration. This reinforces the person-centred value that we are 'a non-coercive companion rather than a guide or an expert on another's life' (Mearns, Thorne and McLeod, 2013, p.2).

Through awareness, then, the roles transcend:

- Persecutor becomes the **Challenger** who is firm and fair in alerting people of the consequences of their actions, and able to assert their side of the contract without punishment.

- Rescuer becomes the **Facilitator** or **Coach** who can support and encourage others without rushing in to solve other people's problems or feeling pressured to provide answers.

- Victim becomes the **Co-creator**, able to negotiate, initiate committed action and connect with self-worth.

Now return to the professional role descriptors you noted above. Has anything changed as a result of becoming more conscious of the drama triangle roles and how they transcend?

ROGERIAN CONDITIONS

For Carl Rogers, the central truth is that the client knows best (1961). If we do nothing else, connecting consciously to Rogerian core conditions means that no harm will be done. These conditions are simplistic in one way, but incredibly profound in others, as they are a way of *being* – when we have unconditional positive regard, empathy and congruence, we accept the core person.

Mearns and Thorne state that a frequent mistake 'is to try to work it out too much in advance. While this feels safer, it puts the counsellor too far ahead of the client and can sound too powerful' (2013, p.111). Instead, equal exchanges are fostered if we engage with our own experiencing, and use intuition to express the thoughts and feelings when they are still emerging. This 'personal resonance' (2013, p.111) draws not only on experience in human communication but also in the professionalism to stay closely attuned and invite the client to respond in as facilitative a way as possible.

Barbara (SLT): My overall focus is to help people develop their confidence in being totally themselves. I listen. Deeply listen. And offer clients an understanding and technical work according to how people choose voice and expression as they wish to. It's a simple thing but so powerful just to be, and listen to people. That's how you start the process.

Active listening means we listen not with the intent to reply, but with the intent to understand (DiLollo and Neimeyer, 2014; Shewell, 2013). We let go of the sense that there is a fixed map of the territory; stepping stones are pointers on the path and the journey it is own destination.

Gwen (E): You have to take a one-toe-at-a-time journey, and that helps you take the plunge eventually, one toe at a time. It helps me manage imposter syndrome.

Annie (V): Trans voice and the kind of self-reflection involved makes it an opportunity for the speech and language therapist to go on a different journey. It's a very unique opportunity.

ACCESSING COMPASSION: USING COMPASSION FOCUSED THERAPY

Due to the marginalization of trans and non-binary people, there may be significant experiences for some of minority stress (Meyer, 2003), stigma and complex shame. Shame is a profound and painful sense that someone is fundamentally flawed and where the ability for compassionate self-soothing is arrested or blocked (Dundas, 2018). In our experience, there can be for some clients a deep unease at not measuring up to cis-norms and accompanying rooted internalized transphobia. It is important to state that internalizing various phobias and degrees thereof is a human and understandable response to what are held up as normative standards, whatever our identity. Celebrating trans identities, bodies and voices as desirable, whole and of intrinsic value is fundamental (Lester, 2017; Roche, 2018, 2020). Working therapeutically with practices from Compassion Focused Therapy (CFT) (Gilbert, 2015; Irons and Beaumont, 2017) addresses experience of shame and guilt. CFT is multi-focused and grounded in the neuroscience of emotional regulation (describing threat, drive and soothing systems), in how old and new brain interact, in evolutionary theory, and in the quality of attachments and social relationships. Practices help clients and therapist-practitioners develop insight, kindness and compassion through slowing down and taking time. Whilst CFT is secular in its approach, many practices originate from schools of Buddhism. We can engage both in the deliberate practice of meditation and in the practices of mindful ways of being in everyday life (Barker, 2013).

Christina (E): Keep nudging the relationships that matter to you. Have compassion for yourself and others. It's still not perfect but it's so, so different. I am not hiding now.

In individual and group sessions, we have led a number of CFT-based guided meditations and exercises:

- Soothing Rhythm Breathing
- Creating a Safe Haven – finding joy and tranquility in an imagined safe space
- Compassionate Self – imagining yourself to be a deeply compassionate person
- Compassion Flowing: out for others, into oneself from others, and self-compassion
- Inner and outer soothing voice tone of warmth and kindness (Irons, 2019; Irons and Beaumont, 2017).

Amanda (E): It was very important for me to learn to find more compassion towards myself – slowing down, listening to my wise self, a soft warm tone.

Zoe (E): Having compassion for yourself is the key to absolutely everything – dealing with life stress, and when I accept myself, maybe I don't need to change my voice.

Nicky (SLT): It is important to remember we are working with the whole person – and support people on a journey of discovery which is completely visible in all its stages to the public, making people very vulnerable and at risk in many cases. Trans and non-binary clients have distress, not pathology. We speech and language therapists have to expand out from our medical, clinical base knowledge and help people grow their voices, grow their confidence in the context of social risk and shamed perception of themselves in many cases. We need skills in the art of voice, the art of facilitation, the art of managing process, the art of *compassion.*

Nina (E): I remember at a certain point I started to notice that I could hear my 'feminine' voice a split second before I spoke, like a memory, with the pitch I had practised, and it was a warm tone, and gave me a warm, sort of comforting feeling, and when I did speak out, people said it was a nice voice to listen to.

FINDING SOLUTIONS: USING A SOLUTION-FOCUSED APPROACH

Voice and communication therapy may be the first intervention within a transitional journey which encompasses many perceived problems. Integrating a solution-focused (SF) approach into initial conversations can shift a problem focus towards emphasizing the resources and courage an individual already has in initiating change. This strengths-based approach helps to anchor positivity, and to normalize the valuing of 'small victories', within a process of enormous change that charts unknown territories.

Jenny (E): I'm 100 per cent more confident and I don't worry about what my voice sounds like. It is a long road and I don't think a lot of people know what you're up against and the voice was the biggest brick wall until I did individual and group voice therapy. I relaxed a bit more because I found myself, and sessions helped me find my voice

– that to me was the brick wall of the whole thing. Before, I was: 'just stay silent'. On the whole journey, you've got to stay positive.

Jennifer (E): Dissolve yourself from the problem to find solutions.

Growing self-awareness enables more sharing of a person's positive experiences, such as learning about voice dynamics, small successes with vocal practice, and feedback and affirmation from others (which may include simply not being noticed). This provides a vital balance to the enormous challenges of modifying voice and communication in complex social contexts. Shennan (2014) states that an SF approach has now become 'bedded down' as the approach of choice for many practitioners in health, partly due to more proven evidence of its 'usefulness and its usability across many settings' (p.xii). Shennan also highlights that the 'shapeshifting' quality of SF therapy enables therapists to either implement a structured approach or to integrate elements more spontaneously as the helping relationship develops. Tellis and Barone (2016) specify that, with experience, speech-language pathologists are not necessarily conscious of making these intentional shifts and that such counselling approaches become as instinctive as adapting treatment to progress.

The non-directive style of SF stems from Rogers' person-centred approach, and opens up more possibilities, rather than trying to 'fix' voice. This works well with minimizing cisheteronormativity and binary constructs of voice, and in building the confidence to accept a voice that is authentic whilst also learning to flex and sustain new elements. The client is an active agent. Implicit within the SF invitation to consider a preferred future is the concept of resilience, and building skills for future proofing, discussed in more depth in Chapter 4. One important tool for building resilience is the use of 'instances' – times when what is wanted is happening. This term seems to be gaining favour rather than 'exceptions' which tends to emphasize when the problem is not happening.

Questions

The therapeutic process of asking, listening and then summarizing is central to purposeful conversation that explores goals and motivation. Finding useful questions and integrating them around task-focused work helps to maintain responsibility and a focus on self-efficacy that balances the advice and answers of more technique work and practice.

An SF approach encourages therapists to go further in thinking and using language that is useful to clients and will keep them on task. SF practice treats 'every session as if it might be the last' (Shennan, 2014, p.xiii)

In our first book, we highlighted the story of the famous cricketer Ricky Ponting and this remains a useful reminder of integrating strengths-based approaches into voice therapy. As one of the greatest batsmen of all time, Ricky Ponting was once asked how he hit the ball so far. His reply highlighted that instead of focusing on the fielders (the problems), he focused on the gaps between as opportunities. Useful questions keep clients focused on the gaps and here are some examples to stimulate reflection:

ASSUMPTION
An important part of finding good questions is to *assume* small successes:

- How did you manage to be here today?

- What have you already been pleased to notice about your voice?

- So what's been better?

Such questions and invitations to say more can be embedded in conversations about voice:

- I'm wondering how you managed to do that.

- What did you do that helped?

- What else?

- What difference is it making?

CLEAN LANGUAGE
...and to probe answers, terrier-like, using a person's own words:

- How do you know xxx?

- What tells you xxx?

- So others have noticed xxx – what have you noticed about yourself?

PLURAL QUESTIONS

These assume that there is more than one response, and encourage a more forensic self-analysis of broader aspects of voice and social communication:

- What else have you noticed?

- What else tells you that you are more aware of your voice?

Non-judgemental, respectful curiosity has been a well-documented part of an SF approach since its inception (Iveson, George and Ratner, 2012; Shennan and Iveson, 2011). A more conscious therapeutic focus on listening and responding to a person's own responses, and using these to co-construct steps towards a desired future, build the therapist's confidence in establishing a culturally competent working environment.

Hence the use of 'notice', for example in 'What would be the first thing you would notice?' This is neutral in terms of allowing the client to choose their own dimension of description: thoughts, feelings or actions.

EVIDENCE

This gathering of evidence is particularly useful in moving from the more general to the specific in order to hone achievable small steps to success.

The cognitive task of focusing on evidence that will support behavioural change can be given as an initial 'homework' observation: what happens with voice that you want to continue to have happen?

This can be combined with scaling and probing questions.

- Is that something you want to continue?

- Are you pleased about that?

- Was it hard to do that?

QUESTIONS FOR FORMULATING GOALS

This part of the process focuses on what an individual is hoping for.

- How will you know when those hopes are realized?

  - What progress towards those hopes are you already making?

PREFERRED FUTURE

Although the original SF use of the Miracle Question may not be considered as prominently as it was (for suggested words see Shennan, 2014), the process of co-constructing a preferred future remains a cornerstone of initial goal setting in SF therapy. 'The process begins in the future, at the endpoint of the work' (Shennan, 2014, p.19). Goals determined by the client are built from understanding where a person wants to get to, and 'waking tomorrow' can offer a concrete context to help notice the changes. We can help the client to *imagine* that they are already there in terms of preferred voice and describe what it is like.

- How might you notice your voice is at its best?

- What would that voice sound like?

- How might you use it with friends and family? And in other settings such as work?

The use of 'ifs', 'mights' and 'maybes' reflects that the future is always uncertain to some extent.

- How will you know when your voice is there?

- What is the first thing you will notice?

- What else?

- What differences will others notice?

- What impact does this have on your voice?

- What impact does this have on your life?

Key to effectiveness is not moving on too quickly to what would help and what an individual needs to do. Staying longer with description can often feel uncomfortable for therapists who lean towards a problem-solving style, and it takes courage and practice to flex the muscles of minimal prompting to say more:

- What is the first thing you would notice?

- What is the next?... Then the next?

Encouraging clients to tell the story of their day keeps a focus on the concrete rather than the abstract, and to think small, which is helpful in learning to value small changes, and think positively about small victories.

When clients express negative perceptions, therapists can creatively use SF questions to re-focus on new possibilities towards their preferred future, for example:

Client: 'Well, I wouldn't be so frightened of using voice at work.'
Therapist: 'What would you be instead?'
or 'Where else might you feel like this?' or
'How might you take this into other areas of your life?'

'What difference would that make?' is a widening question and one of most common questions in SF conversations (Shennan and Iveson, 2008).

Shennan (2014) summarizes important principles for encouraging more detail when describing a preferred future:

- concretizing

- maximizing client choice in framing their answers

- encouraging sequential descriptions – from the first small signs onwards

- building on the client's answers

- asking what would be noticed rather than what would no longer be

- widening out and zooming in

- asking for tangible and observable details

- considering others' perspectives

- making interactional.

Scaling

Again, readers may consider using scales as part of the bread and butter of co-constructing goals. It is the use of scaling as *change-focused talk*, rather than it being seen as 'assessment', that differentiates it as part of a psychological approach to support management. Therapists and coaches who are able to stay with how an individual has arrived at that point, and deep-dive into what lies beneath the achievement so far, are using scaling as a key SF tool for change.

- What are the differences that are making it a 3 now rather than a 1?

- What might be small signs of further progress?

Changes in behaviour are first order changes. Responses that are expressed negatively can trigger second order change questions, those that focus on coping in the face of significant challenges:

- How are you managing to cope, given what's happening at the moment?

- What helps you to keep going?

As before, repeating the question 'What else?' encourages analytical thinking and more detailed observation of behaviours in different contexts, and provides important information for client-focused goal setting. Therapists' use of plural questions, and directing the individual to broader aspects of their life, ensures greater understanding of next steps when focusing back in on the specifics of voice and communication.

Scaling can then be followed up with:

- Tell me about any of this that you've noticed recently – even the smallest bits.

- What does that say about you, that you can do that?

Documenting any changes noticed helps to surface the 'sparkling moments' that are also part of a Narrative Therapy (NT) approach described below.

Although no longer emphasized as a key tool, the use of *compliments* can be embedded indirectly as part of valuing individual differences, key aspects that are supporting voice change and resilience in managing aspects of transition.

EXERCISE

Construct SF questions for the following client responses:

- I can't seem to get the pitch and bouncing on words when I'm on my own.

- My voice is what it is – I don't really feel I'm going to make any more progress.

- There's so much going on, I've got appointment after appointment, so I haven't practised as much as I should have.

- It's better when you tell me what you think – I can't hear what my voice is supposed to sound like.

SPARKLING MOMENTS AND JOURNEYS INTO THE UNKNOWN: USING NARRATIVE THERAPY

Narrative Therapy fits exceedingly well with trans voice and communication work because it foregrounds the client as expert in their lives, locates problems as separate from people and champions the discovery of alternative stories of achievement in social, political and community contexts (White and Epston, 1990). Importantly, it helps to make visible those partial and invisible forces of normative, oppressive and discriminatory constructs of living. Once the dominant, problem-laden stories are aired and deconstructed, we seek to connect clients to forgotten and discounted skills, values and commitments. This, in turn, leads to the (re-)discovery of 'sparkling moments' (Winslade and Monk, 2007) and resonances in which the client, therapist and community co-witness and thicken descriptions for the new, affirmative paths of resilience and competence. We have found White's work on rites of passage and journeying into liminal spaces fruitful in assisting trans clients to explore, 'migrate' and stay with new vocal identities and positionalities (Denborough, 2014; Mills, 2016; Mills and Gorb, 2017; Mills and Stoneham, 2017; White, 1997, 2007).

Jan (SLT): One of the key aspects of Narrative Therapy I value is that it is optimistic and offers hope opening up possibilities for change. These ways of working offer new insight into looking at problems and may assist people in discovering knowledge and abilities they already have. I'm particularly interested in the broader context that affects people's lives. Narrative Therapy understands and frames people's identities, not in a vacuum or as simple client–therapist dynamic, but in a historical, social and political context, all of which exert influence. People have *multi-storied* lives. Identities are not fixed and so are open to change.

Alternative stories need airing and oxygen. Narrative does just that. I'm particularly interested in conversations that may lead to revisions in personal narratives. One of the ways is to look out for openings to these neglected, alternative stories. It's about liminal spaces or 'doorways' which take you to new territory. As a speech and language therapist and counsellor, I'm client-led, I take a *decentred position*, with no particular intentions or ideas about where we are going in the conversation. Asking questions to which I genuinely don't know the answer is key. Sometimes staying with the unknown can be challenging. I find I might ask a particular question because I have a sense of where the conversation is heading, or where I'd like to take it, but that's really not helpful in the end. For me, it's trusting that those alternative stories will emerge through asking the authentically curious, genuine questions, and ones which people will respond to.

For me, Narrative Therapy opens spaces. It opens spaces in language, moving away from collusion with the normative and *either-or* binary assumptive oppositions, such as, *good-bad, feminine-masculine* or *fluent-dysfluent*. It makes space for injustice to be identified, explored and expressed. Postmodernism and the work of Foucault reveal how we are limited by language and 'the way things are' offering us a way into identifying and challenging these taken-for-granted truths. Narrative ideas and practices have the potential to assist people in discovering alternative ways of being, alternative ways of talking. It makes explicit what is implicit, and encourages a willingness to be open to not knowing where we are going. These concepts have guided and stimulated me deeply as a therapist.

Danielle's journey of vocal identity: 'Navigating the Rapids'

Danielle's ability to stay with difficulty and keep travelling through the highs and lows of her landscape, without choosing to abort, has been very moving to be part of. We reflected together that she has grown in personal, vocal and psychological stature. Take time to look carefully and see in her visuals Danielle's totally personal self-scores of despair (0 to -10) and well-being (0 to 10); her resources of determination, persistence and eye for detail; support of friendship and the group; and obstacles of anxiety, bullying and the telephone. Now she sings in the shower, and offers this message to therapists:

Danielle (E): Travel with your clients on their rivers of life! Help us be who we want to be, not who others want us to be and that way I can find my grit and hold my head up high. Don't be scared to help me.

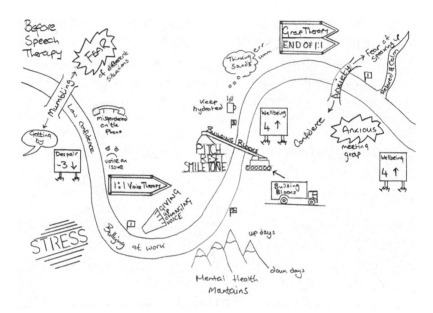

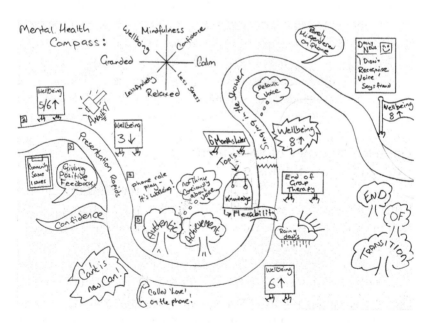

Using therapeutic documents

New stories are fresh, fledgling and vulnerable. The use of therapeutic documents and letters enables conversations to be grounded, and preferred stories to be oxygenated and take substantial, permanent form. They are literary, not diagnostic, and enquire of the client 'what might happen next?' and 'what might be different as a result of finding these new ways of living?' Informal clinical research conducted by White and Epston concluded that clients reported letters as equivalent to 4.5 therapy sessions (Fox, 2003; Denborough, 2014). Documents mark the rite of passage of the end of therapy, such as migration-journey maps, certificates of achievement and words of appreciation, and help clients re-enter their social landscape, not as novices and clients, but as elders and consultants (Epston and White, 1992). Their benefit can be amplified through 'definitional ceremonies' and 'outsider witness practices' in which clients tell and re-tell their stories in front of groups who witness and respond (Denborough, 2014; Leahy, O'Dwyer and Ryan, 2012; Logan, 2013).

1.NADINE'S STORY: 'AS BRAVE AS I'VE BEEN'
Nadine had an initial and therapy appointment with Nicky (SLT). Nicky wrote the following letter to Nadine after the initial appointment.

Dear Nadine,

Thank you for attending the initial consultation with me to discuss voice exploration. I aim to help you explore, create and sustain authentic voice and communication congruent with your sense of self.

You gave me a summary of your transition and clinic appointment history to date. You are about to commence oestrogen therapy and it was good to hear that your GP is supportive.

We spent some time together understanding the current issues in your life and how they may create opportunities or obstacles to your desire to step into a new vocal identity. You told me that your family have struggled with your decision to transition. You are committed to being who you want to be and despite the hostility you have felt, you show courage and strength to 'just get on with it', and work towards your 'exterior and interior self, matching each other'. You have shown the determination to avoid talking situations less and have had the willingness to 'jump in with two feet'.

You work as a chauffeur and have found your line manager to be very supportive of your transition. You told me you have changed your name and you are about to meet with the new boss of the company you work for to explain what has been happening to you, and how you would like them to address and treat you. I wonder how that meeting will go, and how you can use your strength, courage and determination to help you both in that meeting and with your clients?

You spoke of the positive experiences so far of using your feminine voice with strangers, and I would be interested to hear how this develops. We talked together about moments when you might feel better about your voice, and times when you might feel some anxiety.

You were very easily able to identify your hopes for voice and communication therapy. These are:

- 'I want my voice to be softer, particularly when feeling nervous.'

- 'I would like my feminine voice to be a bit higher and sort of brighter than it is now.'

- 'I want to understand how to change my voice.'

- 'I hope to increase my confidence in speaking.'

- 'I want to being able to talk to people comfortably in a calm and relaxed way.'

You were able to tell me about aspects of your communication you currently like, such as – thinking before you speak, going for what you want even when feeling anxious, using a softer voice with strangers, who have responded well, and this has delighted you. You have support around you from your friends and you have found them very helpful in encouraging you to talk up and go for what you want. You have realized that being happy is very important to you and is a strong motive to continue on this journey towards an unknown and unfamiliar place, which may bring up feelings of fear and worry. It may be helpful to keep in mind what goes well for you, to collect stories of success and recruit the supportive people in your life to help you on this journey.

We measured your voice today, with your permission – thank you. You use your voice well and it is a clear sound. We recorded your most frequent pitch as 108Hz when reading and 111Hz when speaking. Everyone has a very individual frequent pitch, and yours are likely to be perceived as typically and traditionally more masculine at the moment by the general public. We will explore what feels authentic for you to explore in terms of pitch change. We discussed that voice involves not just pitch but tone, or resonance – and we can explore the many possible resonances in your voice, to help you achieve what you call a 'brighter, softer' sound. As a listener, I felt very comfortable talking to you and I look forward to further sessions with you, getting to know you, guiding you in this process and learning from each other what works best in order for you to achieve your authentic voice and communication.

You are clearly ready and enthusiastic to start. The therapy try-outs we did together showed you have a keen ear to match pitch, and a flexible voice. We have agreed, then, to begin a programme of exercises to explore pitch, resonance, intonation and voice quality. After individual sessions, you may benefit from voice group which will help you develop your voice skills in more challenging social contexts in a supportive group of ten people in a similar voice process (such as speaking on the telephone, voice projection in noisy environments, public speaking) and build confidence in using your voice in everyday life.

Have a good month, and I look forward to seeing you in our next appointment when we will start 'vocal gym work'!

Best wishes,
Nicky

In the subsequent therapy appointment, Nadine spoke of how it felt to receive the letter.

Nadine (E): It gave me enormous confidence to go forward, and it helped me with my wobble. I felt that you showed a genuine interest in me as a person and I am not like a one-in-one-out-the-door. It is something I can keep reading and go back to. It feels alive and it's really important for me to go back to. It's helped me make my 'trans plan'. The situation is not going to beat me.

2. Sarah Belinda's story: 'Part of the sisterhood'
The following is Matthew's review and discharge letter to Sarah Belinda.

Dear Sara Belinda,

It was really good to see you in the voice sessions and hear both the things you have been struggling with and your stories of achievement.

You told me, and the other group members, that you enjoyed the individual sessions, their quietness and focus, and that it had been challenging after the first group session. You told us that you felt the other group members were 'further on' with their voices, and that you were worried that you didn't have 'as developed skills'. You were feeling 'not good enough' and that you were 'taking up time', and you said you spoke of not returning to the group, perhaps.

I was really struck that you did return, and came to all the sessions, and I wondered – what qualities in you were enabling you to do this? You told us that you found, perhaps re-found, a determination and strength in you to return, and that you had enjoyed the group camaraderie and sharing which was 'really special' to you. This helped you take small steps to being the 'best version of yourself' and having your 'best feminine voice'.

I heard that you found the role-plays meaningful, and discussions about coping with difficult days helpful. You spoke out your feeling of being kinder to yourself and the group heard this. You shared that you were making friends here and finding more confidence to use what you called the 'smile tone smoothness' in your voice.

In our sharing 'check out' in our fourth session, you told us that you were being more spontaneous with your voice, just letting it come out. This has been a journey for you. This resonated deeply with me, because there have been moments in my life when I have felt unable to speak for fear of judgement about my voice by other people, for not sounding typically masculine enough. Your courage to 'grasp the nettle', as you put it, to speak up using your feminine tone and expression fitting you, was heard by the group. Your words filled the room and it was a very powerful moment. I am remembering that in particular, and your courage has inspired me to take more risks with my voice.

In our final session, the 'words of appreciation', group members told you they had been touched by your grace and enjoyed your sense of humour. People said your hand gestures and facial expression are 'utterly feminine' and 'fitting with your voice'. This, you said, was an important moment and feedback for you.

I have really enjoyed working with you in individual and group sessions, and Gillie and Mary have been moved by the things you shared too. I think that you are a very warm-hearted and stylish woman. If you are able to remember the achievements you have made with your voice, and that you are courageous and good enough as you are, I wonder where this will take you next in your life? What differences might this make?

I'm looking forward to seeing you in our review session.

With best wishes,
Matthew

Sara Belinda's response:

Dear Matthew,

I loved receiving your letter! It was very much appreciated, but before I begin to answer it, I want to say something just as heartfelt as any of the points I will be making: when I left the last of the group sessions – and because I had come to enjoy them so much – I felt the inevitable sadness of something having come to an end, and the sense, from that point, of having to fend for myself. (This, I realized, was unavoidable, because, after all, and for practical reasons, no course of therapy can go on indefinitely.) But what I soon realized is that I had taken in more than I had realized, and so fending for myself was a little less problematic than I had perhaps anticipated. To explain, during the group sessions, I sometimes felt, in spite of my dark-haired presentation (that is one way of describing a wig!) like the dumb blond in the room(!), notwithstanding the support I was receiving from yourself, Gillie, Mary and the group members, but obviously (as I quickly, 'post group', realized) I had stored quite a lot of information subconsciously (to add to what I consciously remembered) and the sub-conscious information kept resurfacing in my conversational encounters away from the clinic.

I will now answer your letter, I hope, by describing where I am at, as a result of growing confidence in using my voice.

The key, for me, seems to be, when addressing any person I encounter, is to be 'unguarded'! For so long in my life (I realize) I had been addressing the tiresome (for me) chore of conforming to a male stereotype that I thought was expected, even required, of me: i.e. somewhat gruff and combative, with a modicum of callousness without being offensive. But it was all, and always, an act: my impulse was to be gentle and kind (albeit, hopefully, assertive when needed). Social gatherings were, as a consequence, always stressful, and I often preferred to find some pretext to staying away. Now, it is as if (as a result of the unguardedness) I am taking life less seriously. (This is also to do with my transitioning journey as a whole.) I feel more light-hearted and this informs my lighter, more carefree, tone of voice. Also, the lighter unguarded tone seems to have found its way into my writing! I write stories and now try to think of this activity as something I do 'for fun', rather than take too seriously (which I probably tended to do before). The more and more I have the sense of being female, the more it seems to 'free up' my writing!

A good way, I found, of being less concerned about being 'rehearsed' when speaking, was to remember that another person's conception of me has to do with my appearance and mannerisms as much as my voice, and this means that I am less shy in using my voice and less worried about always 'getting it right' i.e. being more relaxed about my voice. On the telephone, where my voice has to 'do it all', I have had to speak to many individuals in connection with utilities, banks, loyalty cards, etc. and have become more confident through practice, in speaking in a lighter, livelier tone during these conversations.

I feel happier! Why wouldn't I? I am myself, and possibly for the first time in my adult life. This seems to show in my voice.

You asked me in your letter, Matthew, where I think my progress will take me. Well, I think that I will be able to 'use' myself more effectively – I mean in a sense joining the workplace. I would like to work again, though can't work in advertising any more, but would work contentedly in another field – for example, a shop or store.

Taking part in 'Pride' recently – walking with my LGBT friends behind the Woolwich Metro float – was hugely enjoyable for me. I have seldom, if ever, felt so much 'part of the world', with thousands of people on either side of the road cheering and applauding us as we passed by them. I turned to one of my friends during the walk and shouted to her (with all the noise I had no alternative but to shout) 'I am having the time of my life!' And this feeling of being part of the world extends to when I am out and about, around the shops, or coming into London, and seeing other women around me, I derive a sense of reassurance that I am myself, now, one of the 'female tribe' and part of the sisterhood. That probably sounds a bit grandiose a way of looking at my situation, so to bring it down-to-earth, so to speak, I feel the comfort of knowing that I 'belong', and hopefully am accepted as female. I ask for little more than that, really, so it was an unexpected and surprising bonus to find such words as 'elegant' and 'graceful' used in respect of me. But I will shamelessly accept such descriptions and try to live up to them as well!

With best wishes,
Sara Belinda Brown

Matthew's response:

Dear Sara Belinda

Thank you for your letter and such care in your words. As I read and re-read it, I can hear your voice – speaking out – the new unguarded you! It sounds to me like you are more than fending for yourself, and I am moved to hear your joy in belonging in the sisterhood. I can imagine you in one of the Pride pictures, rainbow flags and cheering all around, friends sharing, smiling and standing proud together. How will it be to carry on shamelessly in these ways in your life? You sounded free and unguarded on the phone last week when I phoned to confirm our final appointment time, and it reminded me to seize the moment and be free and smiley with my voice on the phone too! Thank you.

See you at the end of the month for our final session.

Best wishes,
Matthew

In the final session, Sara Belinda spoke of delighting in letter writing, words and the precision of language and punctuation, and being able to tell and develop her story.

Sarah Belinda (E): Living shamelessly? Oh, yes. I am no longer playing the role of being female but being female. Instead of visiting the world, I am *owning* the world that I inhabit.

3. Amanda Malovics' story: 'The worm,
the snake and the dragon'
Amanda chose to explore being present when giving a presentation in one of the group sessions. She was able to be with her vulnerability and give a rich description of her life.

AMANDA'S PRESENTATION

My story is about three animals inside me, which are symbols of my life journey. I was the worm, living in the dark, turning away from life, thinking about dying all the time – but the paradox was that I wanted to live, desperately – and so I changed into and became a snake – symbol of someone trying to be strong,

---

rising up and understanding myself, taking responsibility for myself, moving to London from Budapest, the snake means I am healing myself. Ever since I moved to London and have become the snake, my self-confidence has become stronger and stronger – the snake 'period' is about learning: I am learning how to be my own authentic feminine self, how to express myself. The snake period is the most authentic part of my journey – where I have grown up and learned how to take care of myself, how to make my own decisions, how to be responsible for them, how to find ways to build myself up. Eventually, the snake will become a dragon – representing freedom and power. I am sometimes becoming the dragon, confronting and defeating my fears of being looked at, of having pictures taken of me, of being seen by people and heard by people. I'll become fully the dragon when I make inner peace with myself. My goal in life is to be seen, heard and to inspire and motivate people to be themselves.

In the fifth and last group session, members each contribute to and receive Certificates of Achievements and Words of Appreciation to take away as a group resonance and celebration of themselves.

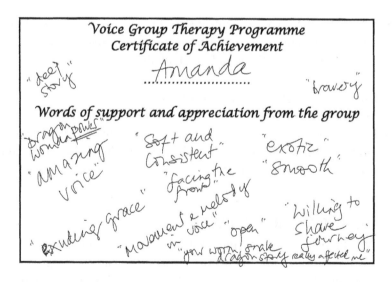

In the final review, Amanda spoke of how it felt it to receive the certificate, and what difference these words made to her.

Amanda (E): They are like treasure. It was touching, so lovely that people gave me their words of encouragement for the things they thought I had done well with my voice, or just about being me. It was something special to take it home as a record, a certificate – something fun too – caring about each other. I am really open about being myself and people knowing that I am transgender woman but I don't always want it to be the first factor people think about. I have a lot of self-criticism inside, and the group helped me feel more powerful and made me soft in my judgemental attitude to myself, and gave me more push to continue what I am doing – voice related and my own journey of life. I heard other people's stories – and I began to believe what people were telling me about myself. Warm, exotic, feminine voice. Thank you! We all have the same root, and we become our own individual flower. I am fighting for my best life every day.

PAUSE FOR REFLECTION:
Now you have read Danielle's navigation through the rapids, Nadine's bravery at facing challenge, Sara Belinda living shamelessly, and Amanda fighting for her best life, what might be different for *you* as a result of having read these stories?

- How have you been moved?

- Is there anything that particularly resonated with you and your life from their stories, something that you may have done in the past?

- What will you take away with you, and how might hearing these stories make a difference to your professional life and practice?

THE POWER OF NOW: MINDFULNESS

Zoe (E): Mindfulness – it's kind of available to everyone right now – it's so easy to be rushing around and dealing with the hustles and bustles of life in London or a big city, it's easy to internalize the stress and can be hard to stay collected. I think just noticing that makes things change – that's being more mindful, I think.

Segal, Williams and Teasdale (2018) hypothesized that mindfulness training could help people to work with the mind states that drive vulnerability. We include a brief summary here to ground discussion of how mindful breath and body work is integrated into both individual and group work with trans and gender diverse people.

Feldman and Kuyken (2019, p.14) summarize three aspects of mindfulness:

- a state of being present that is embodied and experiential

- a process of unfolding moment-to-moment experience

- a faculty, or trainable quality, that can be cultivated and applied in our lives.

We have already touched on how working with trans and gender diverse clients, many of whom experience overwhelming negative thoughts and perceptions about themselves and their voice, requires the competence and confidence to be mindful of *our own* thoughts, habits and distractions. Anchoring breath and body 'with a sense of interest and care' (Feldman and Kuyken, 2019, p.9) can help both clinician and client to become more present and develop the open, non-judgemental curiosity that is integral to the SF and NT approaches described above. Slowing down perception supports the facilitation of useful questions. Mindfulness helps with self-regulation to sustain and switch attention, and with being more curious, open and accepting of experience (Barker, 2013; Kabat-Zinn, 1990, 2016).

The process of letting go and building trust in both the therapist and the therapy requires understanding of habit and the effort involved in re-patterning. Stepping out of automatic pilot in this way helps with identifying automatic scripts that feed anxiety around social threats and negative beliefs about the self in relation to voice and communication. In transferring skills, letting go of aspects that do not serve well-being can support management of the anxieties and expectations that can paralyze performance in social interactions. Individuals will often come with well-formed habits of scanning information in social settings in order to take rapid action to perceived threats. A more mindful approach that slows thinking and orients attention allows evidence to be examined in more depth and detail, and then played with before taking action. Not only does this gap between stimulus and response open up more possibilities for new thinking, but it also brings awareness of the cognitive load required to process and put new vocal behaviours into practice. 'Checking in' with present states such as fatigue, anxiety or competing demands can highlight why vocal performance differs and the challenge of multitasking in vocal situations.

Mindfulness involves sustained effort but with an attitude of self-compassion that can bring experiencing that is freed from habitual, automatic routines (Teasdale and Chaskalson, 2011). Mindful exercises that encourage switching of attention through auditory, visual and sensing modalities, and from thoughts to feelings to images, can be useful in playing with aspects of voice, and with imagining what the end-goal functional voice feels and sounds like. This has its roots in cognitive therapy and, in relation to trans voice work, these aspects might be expanded thus:

- **Bodily sensations**: mindfulness can create an awareness of tightness or stress that may be generally part of social anxiety, avoidance of using voice, or may accompany attempts at new and, as yet untried, vocal behaviours.

- **Emotions**: letting go of shame, embarrassment and fear enables a more playful, experimental approach to voice. As therapists, we model imperfection, which is important in normalizing perceived 'mistakes' and self-consciousness, and acceptance of vulnerability.

- **Thoughts and images**: identification of mind-wandering and distracting thoughts can highlight when these are not based on fact, and when assumptions are getting in the way of openness and curiosity.

- **Behavioural impulses**: awareness of fight, freeze and flight impulses in social situations, and the link with vocal constriction, speech avoidance and maintenance of habituated voice is an integral part of our SLT work. A more mindful approach opens up the space in which experimenting and more choice of behaviours can be actioned.

- **Plus context**: Azul (2015) highlighted the importance of exploring *vocal situations* in his research into transmasculine voice. Greater awareness of how voice is optimized within a mindful approach brings understanding of what impacts on performance, including others' perceptions, and is expressed eloquently by many of the experts by experience in this book.

BEYOND THE WORD: IMAGERY AND ARTS PSYCHOTHERAPY

We have used image work and an arts psychotherapeutic approach to facilitate trans and non-binary clients' reflection on progress and process. Connecting to image for some enables access to the unconscious feelings and can be liberating. We have a blank canvass and a thematic starting point to explore, and invite clients to share afterwards guided by gentle, mindful enquiry. The 'triangle' created between the image, client and therapist creates a holding for narratives to be explored safely, if the client wishes (Hughes, 2016; Malchiodi, 2012, 2018; Moon, 2016).

Catherine (SLT, AS): When working with people with communication problems, I found myself trying to counsel people with aphasia, developmental disorders, dysfluency, and so on. Trying to give them a voice when they had communication challenges, I realized I was using the channel that they find most difficult – verbalization, speech, words. I subsequently trained as an arts psychotherapist – what I particularly value about it is the silence, and the emergence. Through arts psychotherapy I have learnt about the importance of silence, the importance of allowing things to emerge. As a speech and language therapist, I have worked by stimulating, modelling – filling in, bringing out – all useful, but I have come to understand the importance of the presence, the essence of the person, and giving them undivided attention, being in the moment with them. Image making, I believe, is an unconscious process, and there are many levels – it can be metaphysical – taking us beyond the moment. Through using the image making – maybe just lines and patterns, it can help to contain something, or some thoughts, or it offers the chance to externalize inner feelings. The image making can allow them to just be and find a relief from intrusive thoughts, for example. Or it can be a way for someone to explore. The more I have worked with the image and the art form – using different materials, clay, sculpture, digital art – the more I realized the power of the process. There are many instances of abuse that I witness in my role as an intermediary/communication specialist, for example, where people's feelings have been hidden for many years, pushed down, and it can take a long time for trauma to be processed enough to move to language centres.

Once someone came late into a session, and drew one long red line and one short green line and then in the sharing proceeded to tell something incredibly significant about her life and a major event, which was represented in the image. So, image work stimulates and releases – it is a neurological process, a body process. We know that trauma is stored in the body and we know that Broca's and Wernicke's centres shut down as a response to trauma, evidenced from PET scans and MRIs. When someone is allowed to *move* and *work physically* with the paper, paint or craft material, i.e. *tearing up* the paper or *pouring out* through paint, there's an *embodiment* involved, rather than trying to think of the words, or recall and sequence events. When we are working with materials, we are tapping into those sensory associated memories (SAMs) and allow these unprocessed memories eventually to be processed in a verbal way. It enables people to verbalize in a very direct way connecting them to their feelings. Words can hijack us away from the essence.

I believe the image meaning and interpretation can only be given by the image maker. The image making is a process and not about creating a finished product. It is all about *allowing process to happen*. There is no good or bad. There are many different ways, forms and uses. For trans voice, there may be an element of change, exploration and release, and there may have been underlying shame – exploring the past journey and forming new constructs lends itself so well to art form. You can use themes – 'inside, outside', 'past, present, future', 'certainty, uncertainty', 'beyond the binary' – or people can work with a blank canvas. Our life experiences can cause fragmentation of the self which happens through the knocks, the ups and downs. Through the image and art materials, we can work towards wholeness, integration, acceptance and the place of peace. We can only hope to make the unbearable more bearable.

We invited clients to explore image related to 'voice now' theme.

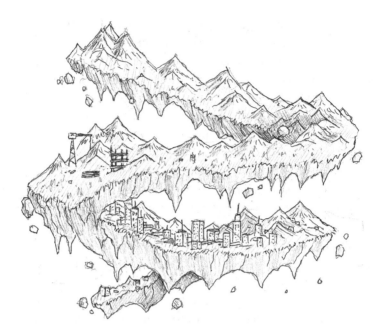

SB shared that her image is 'rocky', 'voice in the world' and that 'it moves, a spiral' and it is 'building up'.

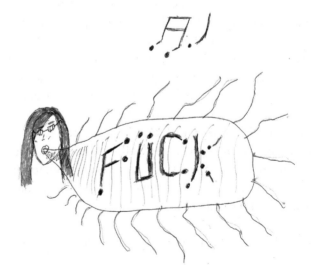

Luna shared that her image means 'protest', 'a tempest for finding my voice', 'I swore my way through therapy', 'my uniqueness', 'own music has to be heard' and 'pink scream'.

CHAPTER 3

The Vocal Space

——— FELT SENSE AND COACHING ———

THIS CHAPTER WILL ASK

What is our experience and understanding of our own voice?

How do we develop relational voice work in vocal coaching?

What is focused clinical practice in trans voice and communication work?

PART I: BEING THE VOCAL EXPLORER

So far, we have examined the lens through which we see gender and how we relate to normative and alternative constructs. We have reviewed what we bring into the therapy and consultation room, the roles we step into, and core conditions we can connect with. We have read accounts of change in action, discovering solutions and journeying into the unknown with clients through a number of psychological approaches. Now we unpack what is involved in coaching and facilitating voice exploration, starting with the invitation to ourselves be the one who experiences and learns about our own voice.

Annie Morrison (V) is an experienced speech and language therapist and voice coach at such conservatoires as the Royal Academy of Dramatic Art, and her understanding and approach to voice work has a deep resonance with identity from physical, psychological and spiritual perspectives. She shares her wisdom here and we draw from a number of those exercises as an invitation to experiment with voice. Use these experiments to re-discover what is simple and what is complex in your relationship with your voice.

What we 'know'

Voice and communication therapy for trans and non-binary people centres client-defined authentic expression (Mills and Stoneham, 2017). The trans voice literature has expanded in the last decade, highlighting collaborative working (Hancock and Siegfriedt, 2020; Mills and Stoneham, 2017); transmasculine voice (Azul, 2015; Azul *et al.*, 2017; Block, Papp and Adler, 2019; Hancock, Childs and Irwig, 2017; Mills, Stoneham and Davies, 2019b; Nygren *et al.*, 2016; Wong and Papp, 2018); transfeminine voice (Davies, Papp and Antoni, 2015; D'haeseleer *et al.*, 2019; Mills and Stoneham, 2017; Oates, 2019); non-binary voice (Mills *et al.*, 2019a); group work (Mills, Stoneham and Georgiadou, 2017; Pert, 2019); service provision and therapist-practitioner competence (Mills and Stoneham, 2016; Mills *et al.*, 2018; RCSLT, 2018); voice and communication with adolescent and young trans and non-binary people (Davidson *et al.*, 2019; Waller and Penzell, 2019). More than knowing this diverse literature and evidence base, the useful, responsive voice therapist and vocal practitioner need to develop their understanding of context and their positionality in the work (Boston, 2018). This, partly, enables us to call ourselves specialist in trans and non-binary voice.

Trans and non-binary people do not have a disordered voice because they are trans and non-binary. There is no mass or lesion on the vocal folds as a result of being trans. There can be, though not always, high levels of social anxiety and isolation, and degrees of conflict over speaking out, at times realized as laryngeal constriction but not often converted into psychogenic dysphonia. Suspected dysphonia warrants an Ear, Nose and Throat (ENT) referral and diagnostics, so that voice can be rehabilitated, if needed, before voice exploration resumes. Laryngoscopy at an ENT or joint voice clinic prior to voice and communication therapy or coaching is not appropriate or trans affirmative, unless vocal pathology is suspected.

Nina (E): Trans is not broken and my voice is not broken.

A referral for voice and communication therapy from a general practitioner, a speech and language therapy colleague, or self-referral in private practice is sufficient. We have already considered in Chapters 1 and 2 the history of medicalization of trans healthcare and how it is essential to reframe our interventions in this field away from diagnostics and assessment-based voice disorder formulations. Pearce (2018) states that trans and non-binary people ought not be subject to more layers of interrogation and burden of proof or diagnosis than cis people. Some general practitioners may need awareness training in the issues discussed here.

Annie (V): I am genuinely interested to know what makes speech and language therapists or pathologists qualified in a field which is not about pathology. Maybe in this field you need to go and do some voice training, because that is where you are going to find your own vulnerability about what your voice is and is not, in support of someone who exploring voice related to their identity.

Singing and voice training in the nineteenth century evolved into theatre voice pedagogy from the early twentieth century and voice science some half a century later. As a result, these fields share the same theoretical underpinning and principles of healthy and expressive voice production (Boston, 2018). Whether voice therapists or voice coaches-practitioners, we share a pedagogical corpus and tradition, joined by an intention to facilitate and give voice – what Bonenfant identifies as 'a vocalic body' (Bonenfant, 2010, p.76).

Positionality: 'being in the boat together'

In the absence of rehabilitating vocal pathology, then, we accompany our clients on a journey of discovery into the unknown. It is, as it were, an archetypal journey to the new world and we, like Jason and the Argonauts, navigate uncharted waters, seek to slay the hydra and claim the golden fleece. The therapist and coach is the companion-hierophant who offers some guidance, but holds no fixed map of the territory. In accompanying the client on their vocal quest, we cannot stay on land *and* make the journey; we have to be on board, in the boat together, casting off together.

Annie (V): We have to cast off. And taking knitting as an analogy and meaning of casting off, if we are existing in the fabric of our life, we are going to drop a few stitches and the therapist has to feel confident about taking risks and letting go of being the expert.

'To cast off', from the Norse *kasta*, means to set free.

Clients arrive at an initial appointment as experts in their own voice and self-concept. Being on board in the process necessitates that we acknowledge our vocal fears and embrace our own lived and explored vocal experience. We are able to hold a considered position within and beyond cisheteronormative vocal constructs, and offer up our vocal skills and limitations for the client's exploration.

Annie (V): Being able to hold creative tension within oneself is the place where you meet other people holding creative tension in themselves – and that's why in this kind of voice work you need to be psychologically aware. If you have not met within yourself those conflicts and how you get warring bits of you to talk to each other, how can you facilitate that for others? If we put ourselves forward as 'I am all worked out, I don't have any conflict', that just means we haven't lifted the lid!

Acknowledging anxiety about our own vocal 'performance' and 'profile' is reflexive practice and therapeutic congruence in action. When we are psychologically and vocally congruent our voice has the ring of truth; clients know and feel it.

Maggi (V): As a I psychotherapist, I knew that I had no right to sit in this chair (as a therapist) unless I had sat in that chair (as a client). It's the same for me as a voice coach, and especially in my work with the trans community. I need to have an inner experiencing of knowing what voice connection is – otherwise how can I communicate what it is to the people I work with?

Sasha (E): My experience of voice therapy is that it has been client-led and the approach has been that therapists are learning stuff too. I think that's a really important attitude.

Vocal experiments and enquiry

Annie (V): When I was training to be a voice coach, having worked as a speech therapist for several years, one of the assignments, one of the experiences I had was of working on a piece of text, speaking out a poem. And I was feeling very vulnerable about it because I hadn't had any actor training. So, I didn't know how to do this 'thing'. All I had was my voice – which I thought was full of flaws, I didn't like it, it was embarrassing, I don't really like performing, don't like being looked at – so I felt very exposed. And having said that, I absolutely love poetry and have always read poetry to *myself*. So, that's the trouble, when you are speech and language therapist, going into a what might be construed as more of a performative space, or being put on the vocal spot, as it were, for many, it can be very unnerving or threatening.

In a fast-paced world that prioritizes delivering projects and achieving outcomes, we may rarely take time to make an unbreakable appointment with ourselves and listen to the wisdom of our body. Immersing ourselves in our vocal learning gives us that time – to notice, sense, re-connect and re-member. We are able to engage in the alchemy of our vocal performance and develop complex and holistic connections through play and practice (Bogost, 2016; Hogan, 2018). The knowledge gained is wholly complementary to our preferred therapeutic approach and practitioner pedagogy to facilitate the optimum voice production, as, for example, Estill (Steinhauer, Klimek and Estill, 2017); Lessac-Masden Resonant Voice Therapy (Verdolini Abbott, 2008); Stemple's Vocal Function Exercises (Stemple and Hapner, 2014); semi-occluded vocal tract exercises (SOVT) (Titze, 2006; Titze and Verdolini Abbott 2012); performance and teaching voice and public speaking (Berry, 1994; Carey and Carey, 2008; Houseman, 2002; Linklater, 2006; Martin and Darnley, 2004; Nelson, 2017; Rodenburg, 2015, 2017; Shewell, 2009).

The experiments that follow are designed to (re)awaken self-awareness and centre your vocal discovery, before scaffolding that of clients. Take your time with them. Embrace a compassionate, mindful approach to let go of automatic judgement and muscular armour that serves to protect and defend. Somatic wisdom and the vocalic body that comes from being human will then emerge.

EXERCISE: Mindful preparation for experiments

Use your own preferred mindful practice, or follow the sequence below as preparation.

- Take a moment simply to sit and be.

- Allow yourself to experience a 3-minute breathing space (an awakening, gathering, expanding practice) where you are sitting now, to bring softness to posture and be open to possibility.

- Plant your feet. Close your eyes or let your gaze soften and de-focus.

- Check in with yourself how things are now: notice body, sensations, thoughts, feelings.

- Bring your focus gently to the breath.

- Be curious in noticing the pattern of your in-breath and out-breath, moment by moment.

- Notice where the breath enters and leaves your body.

- Notice your body's response to breath: the gentle rise and fall of your chest and abdomen.

- Notice when your mind wanders, which may happen many times and that is okay as that's what minds do, and gently bring your attention back to the breath.

- Become aware of yourself as a whole person within your environment.

- Notice the sounds in the room and those outside.

Allow this alert, soft presence to be with you as you work through the vocal experiments...

Annie (V): It's about being able to *be* first before you can *do*. The reason why any vocal experiments need to be as simple as possible is because this work is complex. Human beings are very complex. So, by making them very simple you are re-establishing a primal relationship to the world.

Experiments offer ways of interrogating a part of our body – letting go of the jaw, unlocking the knees, releasing the tongue root, allowing the free breath, exploring resonances. Allow your self-talk to be encouraging with a tone that is warm. Be open and curious: we may discover more by choosing to engage with what emerges.

EXPERIMENT 1: Claiming your standpoint in the world

- Remove footwear, if practical, and let your feet be in sensual contact with the ground with your feet.

- Move from sitting on a chair, or on the floor, to standing.

- Ensure your feet are hip-width apart, knees are unlocked and your neck is free.

- Stand tall and look around you.

- See out to this horizon line.

- What vantage does standing give that sitting did not?

- What arises in you from allowing your eye line to be towards the horizon, to see the overview, to claim this standpoint?

We have absorbed into the unconscious those first moments of negotiating gravity in standing upright. In that first experience, the child has an enormous sense of suddenly having a standpoint in the world. They are able to move with arms free, as an agent of will, with the perception that world is in service to them for satisfaction of their needs. The socialization that follows rapidly means we begin to construct an ego to have those needs met, somehow, and we find creative and adaptive ways of doing so. These end-gaining strategies, though, have reduced us in some ways because constructing an ego is a sacrifice of some central part of who we are. This partly explains why many people tend not to like the sound of their own voices. We have voices that have been constructed by life and what we have had to enact to meet its demands. Therefore, finding the primitive, free sound – that is there in all of us and comes from owning our standpoint, is such an important first step. When we claim, and re-claim it, we relate to our core and our potential. Thereafter, we can consciously explore flexible and diverse constructs to meet life's challenges, express our uniqueness and maintain our safety.

Annie (V): In ourselves we are ourselves, we are us. You are standing up as yourself – coming into your power. You can see over it, over there. When you are getting into your standpoint it is a fresh start, a fresh opportunity for you to feel yourself standing in space as *you*, regardless of where on the continuum of gender you are.

Early in voice exploration we may feel we have to tell ourselves or our clients to breathe. No we don't have to, our body breathes, our body breathes in – our body keeps us alive, there's an agenda there, life coming through us. It's actually very hard to die. Giving voice means we are dealing with paradox – everything related to the voice involves paradox – and that means we are really dealing with truth at a deep level. So, one of the first enquiries, which is so simple but can be mind-blowing for people, is to bounce on your heels breathing out.

EXPERIMENT 2: Bouncing on your heels and breathing

- Work barefoot and enjoy the contact with the ground.

- Stand up and take your standpoint again.

- Start with bouncing on your heels, and breathing out as your heels touch the ground.

- Notice how that feels and how your breath moves in your body.

- Bounce on your heels again, this time breathing in as heels touch the ground.

- Notice how that feels and how breath moves in your body. What changed?

Probably you found it more restrictive to bounce and breathe *in*. We fill up with air and are unable to release. This simple physical action reminds us, and those we work with, that we can let go of the false sense that we have to 'do breathing'. We know about and experience elastic recoil. When clients are distressed and anxious, wishing for quick fix and salve, real alleviation of distress comes from slowing down and taking time to explore the synergy of natural breath flow and body connection mindfully.

Annie (V): The way the wiring is set up, division into voluntary and autonomic nerves controlling striated and smooth muscle respectively, reflects a distinction between the management of internal life and external interaction with the world. The vagus is especially important here because it mediates between the two. It intimately links the gut, heart and larynx. We have those involuntary vocalizations that happen when there's fight flight response to attack – we get the noise – the scream, the roar – that is not you consciously roaring; the roar is coming from your body's place below the waist. You don't have time to think about taking a breath, yet the body breathes. We've learnt to inhibit spontaneous responses, breath is shallow and we assume responsibility for filling up. We are split from ourselves. In Iain McGilchrist's book *The Master and his Emissary* (2009/2019) he talks about how split off we are becoming.

EXPERIMENT 3: Big toe touching down

Renew and explore your sensual connection to the ground – barefoot if practical.

- Stand with your feet hip-width apart and release you knees (tighten your thigh muscles then release them and you will notice your patella move forward).

- Stand on the tripod of both feet – your weight evenly distributed through the balls and heels of your feet.

- Spread your toes and allow them to make light contact with the ground. They are part of grounding us, but not by gripping or pressing.

- What do you notice happens to your spine, neck, jaw and breath when you touch down with the big toe?

Practitioners and therapists are familiar with the concept of 'grounding' – feeling rooted into the ground, with skeletal and spinal alignment that allows for optimal, synergistic breath to give voice. Often, we assume we are grounded, without having or re-membering the sensation of what that actually feels like. Body weight may be travelling predominantly through our heels – notice this in the experiment – and this simply means the jaw is activated. It is fundamental in voice work to experience that when our weight is back on our heels, we engage our jaw and our root of tongue. That is the set up and response to gravity. The jaw, the agent of will-power, is preoccupied with *doing* and becomes easily over-involved. The tongue root, the agent of editing ourselves for public consumption, is concerned with protecting and monitoring. Together the jaw and tongue join forces in order to guard our innermost sensitivity, hide our vulnerability and inhibit vocal 'wobbling'. They ensure that what comes out of our mouths is right, appropriate, the good sound, the right sound, gendered enough, and that it 'ticks the boxes'. The moment we gently engage our big toe to the ground, without gripping it, we change this set up: we connect with our centre, the jaw releases and the breath drops into our abdomen. This enables us to 'speak from the heart'.

Annie (V): It is literally jaw dropping and I am just passing that on. And I could see that in the workshop with the speech and language therapists – it was a light bulb moment.

This experiment makes conscious that which has been forgotten in the melée of life, and which will become more immediately accessible through conscious exploring. In time, with motor learning, your big toe will connect without you directing it consciously. You will hear the body connection in your voice, and connect with the readiness to give voice, and you will recognize that you have ceased to be simply a walking, talking head.

How can we disengage the jaw?

Annie (V): The jaw loves attention and people can get over-fixated on releasing it, yet still have it snap back into action the minute they start to speak. Also the tongue can remain tense compensating for lack of abdominal/thoracic breath support, so relaxing your jaw is only half the story. The upper mandible and the structures behind your face (palate, nasal pathways, sinuses, ears and eyes) are portals for our senses. In the West we tend to think of them as passive, yet they actively affect our voice and speech. We may desensitize them to dampen feelings of exposure and protect ourselves from hurtful judgement or, put another way, our jaw has simply taken all our attention. Either way you are unable to speak out freely, because your voice is seriously devoid of authentic feeling.

The jaw requires an awareness of what it is to be too held and what is engagement enough. The jaw is indeed active in speaking – it is an act of will to speak. Focusing away from the jaw to the mask of the face has the effect of keeping it out of the speaking business and jaw-locking the sound.

EXPERIMENT 4: Enlivening the mask

Sit comfortably on the floor or in a chair, barefooted if practical.

EYE POINTS

On both eyes and at the same time. Points may be tender – use firm, light touch.

- Using the tips of the thumbs, press firmly but lightly into the crevice located at the upper inside corner of eye socket and massage in tiny outwards circles towards the ears.

- Using the tips of the index fingers, repeat in the tiny ridge located at the lower middle of the lower eye socket.

- Using the tips of the index fingers, repeat at the lower outer corner of eye socket.

- Using the tips of the thumbs, repeat at the upper outer corner of eye socket.

- Rub your hands together to create gentle heat and cup each hand gently over each eye and allow the warmth to penetrate the eye from the hands.

NOSE POINTS

Use firm, deep pressure.

- Using the tips of the index fingers, press deeply for 10 seconds in the crevices either side of the base of nose by the nostrils, then rub these points.

- Repeat at the midpoint up either side of the nose.

- Repeat at the centre point between the eyebrows with both fingers.

> • Starting from the first point and moving upwards through the second and third points extending into the forehead, rub in a continuous, fountain-like motion, breathing in through your nose as you do this. Do this three times.

Points may be quite tender on first-time contact. Notice any sensation. Palpation stimulates circulation, innervation and lymphatic drainage, and oxygenates areas of our body that have become dull, stiff and disconnected. Some voice practitioners sometimes describe voice as if coming from our belly: what is meant is allowing abdominal movement in breathing to contact our centre so that our voice is visceral and emanates the ring of truth (Berry, 1994).

Annie (V): The mask of the face is the screen upon which your emotional centre, your gut brain, your first brain, the emotional life for what is going on for you, is to be projected – because below the waist, that is your private world – and if we are going to communicate with emotional intelligence, the diaphragm has to touch down onto this emotional space. When you are speaking, you want to have the screen of your face, the mask, showing what is going on, revealing what is going on inside. That's why we can read children – they are transparent – all the hundred muscles in the face are flickering and all the fibres of the muscles are alive, reflecting what is going on with them. Adults learn to inhibit for good reason because to reveal what's going on underneath can be socially difficult.

Activating the nose points stimulates the lungs; activating the eye points stimulates peripheral vision. Stimulating the face points allows the mask to open and the jaw to remain soft. When we engage our mask, we reveal the inner processing, digesting and transforming of our world through the organs of the body. When we allow our faces to express subtlety, what comes out of our mouth is richly and truthfully ourselves and speaks of what is going on within us at that precise moment.

There is a balance to strike. The jaw-tongue duo keeps us safe. It is a coping strategy we have evolved to mitigate social risk. Too much jaw-tongue involvement, though, means the mask is dead and we speak with an 'information-only' giving voice that does not sound deeply invested, and tends to be reduced in range, resonance, flexibility and expression.

We reach for the 'I'm fine' response while our emotional centre is actually churning up and wishing to communicate 'I'm not fine'.

Annie (V): If we are 'living in the attic' only – the cerebral head – it's a good lookout up there – everything is fine, we are not touched, we can disconnect, we can switch things off – we are a talking head and most people don't realize that because of the enormous value placed on knowledge alone. Coming down to the lower floors, as it were, can be quite scary – there may be a few cobwebs – fears of being overwhelmed, and then we realize there's a lot of cost and energy needed to keeping shut off. We speech and language therapists and voice practitioners become trustworthy because all the tiny fuses in the fuse box have become re-connected – so you know that when *you* are feeling something the person you are working with is feeling it: their mirror neurones say, 'oh yes, I am feeling it!' And that can only happen when the therapist or practitioner is in touch with their instrument, able to take risks, and has done some psychological or personal growth work. Otherwise we stay in mechanics alone and there is no investment.

EXPERIMENT 5: Tongue untied
Tongue active projection

- Let your tongue spill out of your mouth like foam from a cappuccino cascading over the top of the mug, and let it hang there.

- Now, stretch the tongue actively right out of your mouth, and after a few seconds, release and let it slowly recoil to the place where it is sitting on your lips.

- Notice the feeling and explore speaking with this loose forward tongue position.

Tongue active retraction

- With tongue tip touching the bottom teeth and lips away from teeth, let your mouth become 'tongue-less'!

- Like yawning, allow the soft palate to lift and the tongue to move right down – keep the tongue tip on the bottom teeth.

- Allow the pharynx to be really open and wide so the tongue disappears from view.

- Repeat two or three times.

With tongue protruded, we access a developmental stage of life where we met the world through sensory, lingual contact. It may be freeing to feel that again; it may feel like we have ripped up the social rule book, like we are being naughty children. Socialization means we literally have had to learn to 'hold our tongue'. In this experiment, we enable a softening of the editor persona manifesting in tongue root and also soft palate – where the gag reflex springs to action – and we can make voice with tongue out. The *retraction* part of the experiment is a particularly strong stretch of the tongue root and soft palate sphincter, and needs be done no more than four times in one session. We also access this stretch in a genuine yawning, making sure the tongue tip keeps connected to lower incisors. Having performed this, we may discover that velar sounds are freer and more focused because the tongue root has regained its elasticity from stretching out stiffened fibres.

EXPERIMENT 6: Sensuality of the lips

- Give yourself permission to pout and pucker your lips as though blowing kisses.

- Speak out the following words slowly, with relish and exaggerated lip-rounding where the vowels allow for this:

    - lustrous, luscious, voluptuous, sensuous, juicy, ravishing, poire (French for pear), Poirot (name of Agatha Christie's Belgian detective).

- Create your own smorgasbord of sensual, 'lippy' words to play with.

Connecting to the sensuality of the lips is auto erotic – our personal, intimate and sensual world. This does not need to be denied or thought inappropriate for ourselves. If we are facilitating this as part of exploring resonance, however, sensitivity is needed for many trans and non-binary people who may experience discomfort in their bodies.

EXPERIMENT 7: Intoning your name

- Sit with your feet planted and your big toe gently in touch with the ground.

- Put your fingers in your ears, so that you are blocking the air conduction and loop-back, and concentrating instead on bone conduction.

- Intone (on a comfortable single pitch) your name over and over again, slowly.

- Notice the phonemic journey, the geography of your name.

- Allow the vibration of the sound to move in your body.

- Notice how this feels and what arises in you.

- Repeat the process standing up.

Some people, trans and cis, grow up feeling alienated by their names for diverse reasons. The sound vibration of the name may feel congruent. Naming at birth may be experienced as an imposition: we are identified and named by a family and a community before we are independently in our standpoint. For some, this can be naming, claiming and shaming. The sensory experiencing of our name in body resonance allows us to discover a personal relationship with it, and *feel* what we do and do not like. Trans and non-binary people may (but not necessarily) change their name as part of their social transition. Using the trans or non-binary person's 'deadname' (previous name) unchecked is very likely to cause hurt and offence. Deadnames are just that: the oxygen, vibration and person's essence has gone from it. People may experiment with different names, and use specific names with particular groups. Intoning our name(s) enables somatic ownership of it (them). It can be entered into as a self-created naming rite of passage.

EXPERIMENT 8: Playing with sound

Play with the many possibilities of your sound colour palette.

VIBRATIONS IN SYNC

- Touch a wooden table, a china cup, a glass bottle, a flower and repeat a phrase.

- What do you notice about your voice in relation to your sensory environment?

MUSCLE STRETCH

- When you wake in the morning, or when you are feeling stiff, stretch out and give voice to that stretching muscle.

STERNUM HOOK UP

- Place the three middle fingers of your dominant hand on your sternum and repeat a phrase, first with mouth closed, then open, and feel the vibrations conducted by the manubrium and sternum to your fingers.

SMILE TONE

- Engage the mask of your face.

- Smile without grinning: imagine you 'have a secret' (on the edge of a smile) and feel the zygomaticus and risorius muscles engage.

- Repeat a phrase and feel the sensation and resonance of the sound in the mask of your face

EAR HONK

- On a 'huh' sound, opening your jaw slightly laterally towards your ear, let the ear emit its own personal 'honk!'

- Repeat on the opposite side.

Playing with our own sound in these ways is beyond any binary. We may initially judge the sounds emerging as not beautiful or tuneful. However, they are body sounds and have intrinsic value, whether they are 'creaking' from stretching, or 'trumpeting' from our ear. The point about ear honking is that this is the sound *your ear* is making and you give voice to it. It opens oral and nasopharyngeal resonance possibilities. 'Smile tone' increases access to the 'bright' resonance of the dome-like skull and 'wide mask' resonance across the cheekbones. When we sense through touch that our voice is 'hooked up' to the sternum, thoracic resonance amplifies, front and back, due to bone conduction by the manubrium and muscular anchoring by the sternocleidomastoids.

We are sentient beings in receiving as well as making sound. Everything is vibrating and we interact with the world's sensuality and soundscape in every moment. We *do* sing more resonantly in the bath because of the ambient acoustics. We may be entranced by the hypnotic and relentless ostinato rhythm in the snare drums in Ravel's *Bolero (it is truly disturbing and meant to be)*; we are subtly, viscerally, tuned to Pavarotti's B4 (494Hz) in Puccini's 'Nessum Dorma' and the idiosyncratic harmonics of Billie Holiday. Whatever our musical taste, we are literally *moved* by coming into contact with these rhythms and frequencies.

Authentic voice

Kermis and Goldman define authenticity as 'the unobstructed operation of one's core or true self in one's daily enterprise' (2006, p.294). It is actioned, relational and dispositional in the way we choose to live life and are perceived as congruent by others (Martinez *et al.* 2017). In voice terms, we have many voices and we code switch all the time to meet social, familial and professional demands. Having a 'telephone voice', for example, is not inauthentic, it is *one* of our authentic voices – devoid of the visual cue, it is our *sonic persona*. Exploring voice means starting from openness, rather than rejecting what is coming out now. When the armoury is removed, new possibilities and fresh perspectives reveal themselves. We may discover and choose to play head resonances more strongly, for example – that is authentic. We are not 'putting on' a voice. Inner listening, not necessarily with our ears, and accepting what is coming out vocally, brings the ring of truth.

Annie (V): For me, authenticity means connection. Connection that comes because the intelligence of the body knows it's being listened to, and it starts to get coloured in. We don't have one voice. The wonderful thing about the vocal folds is that they are fluid – they can get thicker and thinner. How amazing is that! So, playing with the voice through all its manifestations and then exploring your how you want to present to the world – the way you want your person to be received in the world. We are all doing that. For me, I think binary thinking is too limiting. Shades of grey – they are amazing. Shades of white and shades of black – the potential for subtleties and relationships. Humans are complex. So, where do we want to play our music, if you like? Where is the ring of truth if you are trans? Be sensitive to what feels good for your clients, and that is as individual as every individual.

Ultimately, when we move beyond inflexible notions of gendered sound, we are liberated. Here is a set of vocal folds of a certain size, a vocal tract of a certain size, and this is the sound that is coming out now, with many tunes, textures and possibilities (Mills *et al.*, 2019a).

PART I SUMMARY: BEING THE VOCAL EXPLORER

- Be the learner in exactly the same way as we invite clients to be.

- Voice work is an ongoing journey.

- We cannot ask someone to go to a place we have not gone to ourselves.

- We reveal voice by connecting the big toe to the ground, stretching the tongue root, enlivening the mask and playing with sound and its sensuality.

- A voice that is not free is 'put on'.

- A voice that is free is not 'put on' – it is connected, adaptable and expressive.

- Changing voice is a political act; resisting changing voice is also a political act.

PART II: BEING THE VOCAL COACH

Having rediscovered our own vocal potential and readiness to take risks, let us examine in detail the pertinent issues in facilitating a vocal change process for trans and non-binary people. The art of vocal coaching, whether in individual or group settings, involves being able to shift flexibly and consciously on a continuum of teaching and demonstrating at one end, and supporting independence and self-efficacy at the other (Rogers, 2010). Schön's seminal work on reflection in action (1987/2014) highlighted the importance of acquiring both procedure *and* craft. Higgs *et al.* (2008) explore the *art* of being a therapist versus applying rational, technical skills, and it is this artistry that requires us to hone facilitation and integrate coaching skills. Duffy (2015) states that when the facilitator is *in* the work, noticing and experiencing bring a generative approach to facilitation. Being in process with our own coaching and facilitation styles enables us to flex more honestly and responsively between technique and support. We explore this in more depth in Chapter 4 in relation to voice and communication group work. In this chapter, we begin to explore coaching and facilitation in an individual context, where work centres more demonstration, hands-on practice and guidance in establishing the client's process. There may be some tentativeness on the part of developing therapists and practitioners in terms of adapting their known therapy and practice, in order to drill down to the vocal nitty-gritty. We emphasize the principles of motor learning (Titze and Verdolini Abbott, 2012) in the exercises below, and offer some insights into their application to trans voice exploration.

First, at the core is the necessity to be transparent about the potential paradox of voice change. For whom and for what purpose is change sought and desired? Making paradox explicit means we do not collude with pass-fail cisnormative judgements of gender vocal and communicative expression. The more we hold that voice is utterly individual and that it is okay to be trans, the more we move to creating a world which honours the person for being themselves. Supporting people to be human means clients can experience the richness and fullness of themselves to be beautifully, warmly, generously feminine, masculine and non-binary in voice and communication in unique ways. Our role is to be present and explore the parameters of what change is possible, to confront and make visible potentially typical and stereotypical behaviours. Clients may then choose consciously, as we all do, to take on adaptive ways of meeting the world with personal flair: 'The more expanded our definitions, the more space there is for everyone' (Lester, 2017, p.36).

Therapy nomenclature

As we discuss in Chapter 1, terminology is rapidly evolving. As therapists and practitioners, we need to have a nuanced understanding and clarity of what we call the therapy and practice we offer. Our practice has evolved through experience and discussion with community focus groups, such that it is helpful to hold terms voice feminization and masculinization lightly. They are culturally loaded and subjective.

One-to-one sessions witness a huge diversity of clients. Voice group membership includes many clients who are non-binary, fluid, bi-gendered, pan-gendered, genderqueer, non-binary transmasculine, non-binary transfeminine alongside binary trans people. We use affirmative and inclusive nomenclature to support this. Some non-binary people, who do not identify as female, seek to raise pitch and foreground head resonance, so explaining intervention as 'voice feminization' might give offence. Further, we responded to clients' requests to move away from reference to birth assignation. Some non-binary people have spoken of 'queering the larynx'. We aim to de-gender the larynx and use our ears to describe the current status quo of the larynx that arise from actions of endogenous and exogenous testosterone growth process (Mills *et al.*, 2019a).

Nina (E): Ask me 'what do you want me to call this work for you?'

'Voice and communication therapy' and 'voice exploration' are inclusive. Voice modification is mostly benign, but might imply that there is a definite need for something to be modified, when the client may simply want to check that what they are currently doing is healthy and efficient. We recommend starting with voice and communication therapy, and voice exploration, moving to voice modification. Use inclusive language and 'ask' etiquette to see what makes sense for the client in terms of therapy nomenclature.

In the same way, consider the language used in reports. In trans voice, we are not contributing to a diagnostic work-up of a vocal pathology or a formulation towards diagnosis of transsexualism or gender incongruence (see Vincent, 2018). Speech and language therapists and voice practitioners working in healthcare report on current pertinent voice profile and vocal contexts, client goals discussed, and the therapeutic contract, providing colleagues with a perspective on how someone is managing their journey of vocal identity (Mills and Stoneham, 2017) and vocal situations (Azul, 2015; Azul *et al.*, 2017). Clinical letters inform without being evaluative so the initial session may be helpfully recorded as an 'appointment' rather than an 'assessment'. There was a time when speech and language therapists would not see trans people who were not 'living full-time' in social gender role. Gladly, this is now understood as not affirmative practice, since many trans and non-binary people do not seek 'full-time' social role change, may not be able to, may be fluidly moving across gender roles or may reject these notions altogether. As in all therapeutic work, we meet people where they are at, and offer sessions according to our service constraints, working to our redundancy and the clients' self-efficacy. Similarly, it is affirmative practice to avoid such terms as 'fully feminized/masculinized' or grading the trans person's voice against cisnormative standards. Progress can be reported directly relating to client goals. When we analyze pitch with our trans clients, we own that pitch parameter studies are based on cis people and we state the caveat every time as 'typically perceived as feminine/masculine/neutral according to cis norms'.

Nina: I am feminine, so is my voice, in my way, and it had to develop. I didn't want a voice teacher or therapist to say my voice is 'fully feminized' at the end, implying it was rubbish up to then. What does it mean? Is any woman's voice fully feminized or man's fully masculinized? You will mean well but it sounds judgemental, and more about you than me. It's like straight people saying gay people 'turn gay'. Saying fully feminized makes me feel like a recipe and I am not.

Criteria for discharge is based less on attaining a particular sound in a particular way, but in acquiring an accumulation of skills which can be developed further independently by the client.

Lucy (E): Every day is a new day on the voice journey.

When we present our work at conferences and within professional groups, in the absence of our clients, we must be meticulous to tell trans stories with consent and use client language cleanly and in context: 'we continue to be used carelessly by journalists, politicians, researchers and others who feel entitled to take our stories, to make decisions which impact our lives for their own gain, and to get money and recognition on the back of our struggles' (Barker, 2018).

In the same vein, it is problematic to play recordings of trans people's before and after therapy voices. When we listen to voices we may be making unconscious or conscious judgements about how the trans and non-binary person is measuring up to a cis norm. It is a sensitive subject and some clients may not realize the level to which they are seeking passing judgement and approval when they consented to have their voices played publicly. Some non-binary clients may actively seek to take on vocal binary behaviours as far away from birth assignation as possible in order to mitigate the risk of being misgendered and attacked.

Relational voice work

The key element here is the meeting of one voice with another, one vocal profile with another: shared and parallel processing of your felt sense of *your* voice meeting the client's felt sense of *theirs*. This is true of all vocal coaching; it is amplified against the cisheteronormative backdrop where trans meets cis, and cis meets trans. Let us evoke Audrey Lorde again: 'I am who I am, doing what I came to do, acting upon you like a drug or chisel to remind you of you me-ness as I discover you in myself' (1984/2019, p.143).

Mia (E): Really important: you wouldn't ask your clients to do something that you are not prepared to do yourself. It helps trans people feel more comfortable – like you are not just being examined. If the therapist is also making these (potentially) odd, new noises, all the better, it makes it all a bit more fun. Not so nice or helpful if the therapist is sitting there like a stone.

Jennifer (E): Good communication is pattern matching – we pick up and mirror each other.

Following on from your voice exploration above, consider how you would define your habitual pitch and resonance profile.

EXERCISE: Finding your habitual pitch perceptually

Have access to an app or instrument that you can pitch match.

- Count 1–5 slowly and just listen.

- Count 1–10 slowly and now see if you can find the note on the app or online keyboard which corresponds to your spoken pitch on each number.

You will find the pitch on '1' is probably the highest, and then there will be a see-saw between others close by, or a slow descent ranging from three or four notes to finishing at '10'. There will be primary or secondary frequencies (pitches) that you may discern as the most frequent. This is an easy, quick way in to discovering your modal pitch perceptually. Try it out with your friends, colleagues and family as it is a useful skill to practise. It can be used therapeutically as a preliminary step before objective electroglottographic (EGG) measurement, if that is available to you. The exercise gives you information about which frequencies you tend to hit at the beginning of your talk, where you orientate to in terms of mode and where your speaking cadence falls to. Make a note of these related to the keys on the app or programme – *Perfect Piano* is easy to install on smart phones and can be used in sessions, and you can access various online keyboards such as 'Piano Player'.[1] The musical keys correspond to the frequencies in the following table. These are sound-*productive* applications, and you can progress to using any number of useful sound-*receptive* apps which analyze your voice and are available in the market place. There are many useful apps including Voice Analyst, OperaVox, Da Tuner Lite and Eva Pitch.

Musical Note	Corresponding Frequency in Hertz (Hz)
E2	82.4
F2	87.3
F#2	92.5
G2	98.03
G#2	103.8
A2	110.0

cont.

1   www.piano-player.info/

Musical Note	Corresponding Frequency in Hertz (Hz)
A#2	116.5
B2	123.5
C3	130.8
C#3	138.6
D3	146.8
D#3	155.5
E3	164.8
F3	174.6
F#3	185.0
G3	196.0
G#3	207.7
A3	220.0
A#3	233.1
B3	246.9
C4 ('middle C')	261.6
C#4	277.2
D4	293.7
D#4	311.1

Listen to your voice heroes in the media and in life, and tune in to what pitch they are speaking at the onset of their sound.

Mary (SLT): After J.K Rowling, we can seek and find our *vocal Patronus!*

PAUSE FOR REFLECTION: MY VOCAL PROFILE
How would you describe the idiosyncrasies and features of your voice?

- modal pitch and pitch range

- resonances

- voice quality

- articulation

- prosodic character.

In pitch raising work, the therapist-practitioner demonstrating E3 (165Hz), F3 (175Hz) F#3 (185Hz) and G3 (196Hz) needs to be able to explore and explain and the intersections of pitch and timbre between their own and that of their trans female, transfeminine or non-binary client during the process of matching your pitch. When a client seeking to raise pitch hears a cis female production of a pitch at the lower end of the therapist-practitioner range, the client may respond by producing a pitch in a sympathetically lower part of their *own* range. It may be useful, therefore, to demonstrate an octave above the target frequency, in order to enable the client to produce the intended target. It is essential to be able to contrast resonances at the same pitch, for example what a target pitch sounds like with and without facial, pharyngeal and chest resonance. If you are modelling E3 (165Hz) and you are cis female, you are going to experience potentially unfamiliar chest resonance at this low part of your range. You might also experience this as a less focused or powerful sound than that produced in your modal and middle ranges. Simply ensure there is a light but clean vocal note for the demonstration to be adequate. In similar vein, a cis male demonstration of higher than habitual pitch may be perceived by the client as relatively higher in pitch than the frequency/musical note, related to the resonance profile that accompanies the model of the therapist-practitioner. Relational voice work offers creative potential and the means to experiment with pitch and resonance mixtures between the model and the client's attempt, and vice versa.

In the initial stages, your voice model provides evidence that change is possible, if it is sought, and is realized through the reassurance and visual feedback (gestural) scaffolding, masking (where therapist-practitioner minimizes client self-consciousness by voicing over them) and repetition. Whilst potential anxiety and vocal dysphoria are acknowledged early on, new exploration of voice may activate a temporary increase in vocal dysphoria and self-critical, even failure narratives in the client: 'I can't do this'; 'that's weird'; 'how is doing this going to help my speaking voice?' In explaining the *process* and *trajectory* of acquiring vocal competence, we acknowledge risk and mitigate vulnerability.

In exploratory and early sessions, and at times in review apportionments and group choral vocal practice, rhythmic masking and structured turn-taking on the part of the therapist-practitioner helps clients put their 'toe in the water' in order later to immerse themselves in new sounds and sensations:

- counting or clicking the beat: '1,2,3, and go'

- '123 and it's my turn, 123 and it's your turn, 123 and it's our turn together'.

This confident and facilitative structure and shaping – deep listening all the while – is an important therapeutic skill to support and energize practice and make the process safe, and prepare the way for independence.

Nina (E): Voice therapists, SLTs, need to be able to produce a whole range of vocal qualities and play with their voice. The SLT has to *warm up the room* – both in terms of putting trans people at ease by being open and inclusive, and by being confident in demonstrating with their own voice. Clinical or medical rooms can be cold, literally, because of the décor, and because the fear that people may have about being assessed or interviewed. The SLT needs to bring their warmth to the meeting, warm up the room, warm me up, warm up their own voice and warm up mine. That way, I feel safe and comfortable with the therapist and can trust in the process.

Gwen (E): I found it incredibly useful, well it's really essential, to hear the therapist demonstrate vocal exercises, show change, give me a contrast, and let me see the imperfections and potential risk taken by the therapist to help me. It's like we are both mitigating risk by risking together.

As the client becomes more able to self-monitor and take ownership of the work, you can step back from initiating vocal demonstration and praxis, flexibly knowing that re-focusing in a moment of reminder or additional support is flexible coaching without rescuing. As preparation for the session, whatever your gender, go for typically masculinizing and feminizing your own voice, and then playing around with mixing and contrasting, and experimenting between and beyond perceived vocal binaries.

EXERCISE

- Listen to: 'Meet Q – the first genderless voice AI Voice Assistant'[2]
- Can you profile what you hear and copy it?

Review the vocal features you have tried out to date in ongoing voice work and vocal supervision. Practise and enjoy developing this flexibility, so that you are moving beyond your default vocal position and any bias that may be around for you and for the client, that the sound of your voice is the goal.

Vocal transference and countertransference

All relational work, voice included, potentially brings up feelings which the client may transfer to the therapist and which the therapist may, if not conscious and reflexive, (counter)transfer to the client (Mearns and Thorne, 2013). Indeed, countertransference is not always problematic and can be helpful to the client if it is conscious on the part of the therapist. Left unconscious, the difficult feelings triggered in the therapist may 'leak out', and the therapist-practitioner becomes emotionally entangled or enmeshed with client.

How is this relevant for voice practitioners and speech and language therapists working with trans and non-binary people? If you share the same gender identity, cis and trans, as your client, what is being held up as the prized position? If you are cis female, your transfeminine clients will likely transfer feelings that *your voice* is the goal, rather than the *skills* you are demonstrating; if you are cis male, something similar might happen with your transmasculine clients. This is likely to be very unconscious. When a client, subconsciously, desires to embody or sound like a version of the therapist-practitioner, it may feel flattering to the therapist-practitioner but, in fact, it will activate negative reinforcement cycles as described by the drama triangle, ultimately leaving the client feeling victimized for not being cis at all or cis enough. This sort of countertransference, if we are not aware of its mechanism, is seductive as it positions the therapist-practitioner as the one who endows 'passing privilege' to the trans person. Reflexive practice enables us to move beyond co-dependency, and ask questions of ourselves and our clients

---

2   www.youtube.com/watch?v=LLjYccnuFjE

which do not subconsciously elicit answers that speak to the privilege and specialness of the therapist (Redstone, 2004).

Mary (SLT): The number one thing that people say when they come in regardless of gender presentation when we ask them 'Have you tried to modify your own voice?' They say, 'Yes but I felt silly.' All the time. It's so important for therapists and voice specialists to know that and actually go through the process of **changing and modifying your voice yourself.**

It feels ridiculous – and fun – but if I think about using that profile and going into a coffee shop and saying (in masculinized voice), 'Can I get a latte?' It wouldn't sound familiar so it would be weird to do it. The therapist has to go through that empathetic process of I am going to take risk with my voice and really jump in to this, and know how it feels to be using a voice – not putting on a voice – but using a voice functionally in a day-to-day way that is drastically different from the voice that I 'normally' use.

When we are moving to a new 'gendered' vocal position as therapist-practitioner, another layer of complexity enters the process. When demonstrating movement away from your habitual set, you make a similar journey to the client, and feelings of 'imposter syndrome' may kick in – within you and within the client. It may be, for example, that in demonstrating semi-tonal or tonal pitch lowering with increased chest resonance for a cis female therapist, or pitch raising to the region of E3–G3 (165–196Hz) with increased facial resonance for a cis male therapist, the client may hear and reject, subconsciously, the modelled sound for being 'odd' or 'phoney'. When the 'effort' of the unfamiliar is heard in the voice it can register as seeming 'forced' in the first instance. Another scenario: if you are cis male demonstrating a higher starting pitch, there may be some transference around rejecting 'putting on' a typically perceived female voice, which may sound effeminate or camp, and that may be exactly what the client seeks to avoid. Similarly, if you are a cis female demonstrating lower starting pitch and increased chest resonance, the trans or non-binary client may respond with feelings that you sound weak. These scenarios, and other permutations, are the mechanisms of cisheteronormativity at work and vocal gendered normative expectation, and need to be gently acknowledged and made explicit: this is how it sounds from me; this is how it sounds from you. The imposter syndrome is therapeutically useful and part of congruence as it brings the therapist to a lived experience of counter-transferred dysphoria. If it can be owned, it is extremely empowering and permissive for the client. Ultimately, we cannot impersonate another and every voice is beautifully unique.

Carys (SLT): I have to concentrate on my own voice change process. It's continuous, ongoing development. Good to model that. I think I am very aware when I am doing exercises or qualities which 'masculinize' my typical feminine habit voice, this is a very small moment in time for me, and I am doing this 'slightly out of context voice'. That comes down to my own vocal development and pushing my own boundaries. Making my masculine voice sound more connected to me, my 'natural' masculine voice, without it sounding 'put on'. It's really important for we therapists to experience that.

Mary (SLT): When I produce an E3 pitch, that may sound much 'lower' perceptually than it would from a person whose vocal folds have been thickened in first puberty. Making adjustments for that is important, and also being not apologetic but really straightforward about the fact that my cis-ness does have presence in the room and that that is not preferable, that is not a goal, that is the relationship between my voice and me – I have a voice that has been shaped by living in a society where there's an expectation that women's voices will be on the higher side.

Review of exercises in trans and non-binary voice exploration

We offered a number of exercises in our first book and the ones in this chapter are intended as a companion to invite deeper and broader exploration. What follows is a summary of salient points when facilitating binary and non-binary trans voice exploration and a refocusing of key exercises which we feel help you 'cut to the chase'. The regular, mindful practice of exercises is essential – as when learning a musical instrument – but ultimately it is the awareness and freedom the exercises bring that is the objective. Sound is the end result; sensation is the process. We understand an exercise, we try it, we feel it, we hear it, we absorb it. We can offer clients only those exercises we know deeply in our own body.

INTONATION

Perhaps controversially, intonation work does not need to be made overly complex. We have written about *bouncing* on key words in our first book. Intonation is personal and intrinsically linked to our own meaning-making, so bouncing and 'moving the bounce around' is useful in helping clients notice where they are placing emphasis, and developing prosodic awareness. If someone's aim is to be expressive, enable them to enjoy the sensual qualities of words. If we start uncoupling intonation from meaning-making, voice definitely sounds formulaic, disconnected and unspontaneous.

PITCH

In terms of *pitch raising* work, we would say the opposite: this parameter needs to be very specifically identified and practised. We are certainly not placing pitch as necessarily the most important feature to explore, but if a client comes with a goal to raise pitch to feel more congruent, then tackling it head on with very clear frequency targets and movement is the only way forward. If you want your vocal folds to habituate to a faster frequency at the beginning of your talk – the very first voiced sound that emanates from you – with ease and efficiency, you must engage in specific, achievable, easy pitch work that moves stepwise and semi-tonally. Use humming on /m/ followed by intoned (same pitch) rote speech, thinking or hesitation sounds (such as 'err', 'um', 'so', 'well and-er', 'so-um', 'well-er-so-um…'). Below we include a schema of vocal shaping from, where position 1 is the start and onset of the voice, and the place of most consciousness and preparation. Position 2 is the top of your speaking voice and you do not need to worry about what that pitch is, as long your client is not moving into a falsetto voice quality. Falsetto is fine for singing at higher pitches; it is not speech quality, unless you are being playful with 'character voices'. Position 3 is the 'bottom of your speaking voice' position – this may be conceptualized for a binary trans woman, if relevant to the voice exploration, as being 'a new grounded position' as it tackles negative perceptions of a 'voice dropping down' narrative.

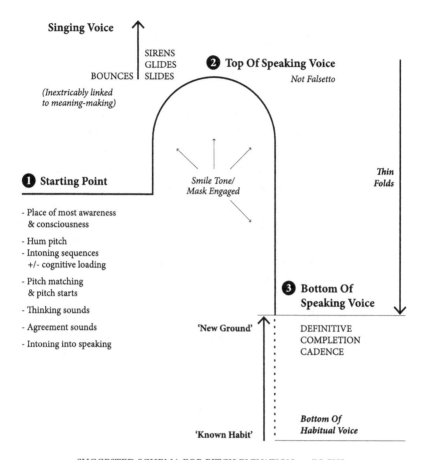

SUGGESTED SCHEMA FOR PITCH ELEVATION ++ FOCUS

Gwen (E): In individual and group sessions, we reinforce our own and learn other people's life hacks! Not tricks, life hacks. Hacking the system – for example, the 'uh-huh' and 'm-hm' and a lifted started pitch – these are fantastic to change voice, unnoticed by others, in conversation flow, and giving those social cues that I am listening, please continue! It's a great life hack! And when I come to speak I already have engaged the right muscles to work to get my voice out as I want it to be.

Lucy (E): Detailed pitch training at the moment of beginning speaking, the very first thing, is essential. And eventually my muscles find that set and become more and more used to achieving it. That also includes hearing it. I am now literally used to my voice and can't recall (internally) my 'old voice' or actually find the way I made it. That's what I did to achieve my voice: speech therapists need to be really on it about what pitches work for me and my personal voice goals, show me (do it), and help me practise it, so I can keep on doing it myself so it becomes a habit, something automatic.

Mia (E): Having a musical understanding as a singer helped me access very quickly in my head and hold within a semitone my springboard pitch, that specific pitch. But I saw evidence of everyone in the group achieving that, whether they were musically trained or not, they tuned in, we all did, and we found our starting pitch we'd been working on. It's a kind of memory a split second before you go to speak. So, I would say to speech therapists that they need to help people learn that skill by being totally pitch specific in the starting pitch – i.e. that very first sound – not generalized, don't just say 'up a bit' – that doesn't me help develop it ultimately.

Stabilizing raised pitch starts with agreement sound 'm-hm' /mɱm/ is very practical and immediately applicable to conversation. What is essential is that in practice, the repetition of the /m/ and the initial voiced /m/ of the 'm-hm' is carefully matched and that the rising inflection on 'hm' does not influence a 'preparatory drop' in the /m/ of the 'm-hm'. See diagram below – the aim is to stabilize.

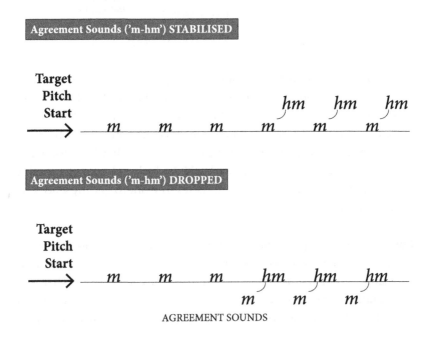

AGREEMENT SOUNDS

In the absence of vocal fold thickening caused by testosterone, *pitch lowering* work is best incremental and subtle – from semi-tone and whole tone, and no more than a whole tone lower than current habitual pitch, otherwise there will be hyperfunction and vocal strain. It is very useful to experience this in your own vocal practice – how low can you go from your habitual pitch without pushing down and constricting?

RESONANCE

There is a literal and symbolic meaning in resonance – to prolong and amplify sound due to synchronous vibration of a neighbouring 'object'; to be in sync and share rich significance with someone. Cicely Berry described resonance as that which draws the listener in to your sound (Berry, 1994). The following is a review of resonance work which you can explore with clients:

EXERCISE: Reviewing 'smile tone'

Used for brightening tone and anchoring sound with zygomaticus major and minor, risorius and nasalis. Note this is not grinning and showing teeth; instead imagine 'having a secret' and engaging the facial muscles.

Use humming with vowel sequences to play with formants 1, 2, and 3.

Starting with 'ee' /iː/ vowel helps to brighten to the tone and generalize brightest to other vowels in the following sequence:

- Repeat 'me' /miː/ three times, then 'meh' /me/ three times, then 'ma' /mɑː/ three times.

- Begin again with 'me' /miː/ three times, then with lip-rounded vowels 'moo' /muː/ three times, 'mor' /mɔː/ three times, and finish with diphthong 'moh' /məʊ/ three times.

Notice brilliance in all vowel and diphthong profiles.

EXERCISE: Reviewing 'sternum hook up'

Used for deepening tone.

- Place fingers on sternum.

- With a comfortably low hum, use chest tapping to emphasizing bone conduction and chest 'placement' of sound.

- Repeat and open to 'ah' and again to 'oo'.

EXERCISE: Re-visiting 'yawn space'

Used to release editor in the root of the tongue to increase pharyngeal resonance.

- Keep the tip of the tongue in contact with the lower teeth, and ensure vocal tone is not breathy when generalizing the sound into speech.

- Explore 'ah' and sequences (days of week, counting, etc.) with exaggerated yawn talk.

- Repeat naturalistically aiming not to sound like yawning but keeping the kernel resonant space and sensation and a softness at the back of the tongue.

EXERCISE: Revisiting 'across the space'

Used to develop 'squillo', 'blade' or twang voice quality.

- Explore your preferred variations of quacking, cackling, and the sound the aliens make in the film *Mars Attacks*.

- Use 'Hey!' and 'Hey you!' and throw the sound to someone across the room. Ensure that your tongue is high in your mouth and engage smile posture.

- Ensure the sound travels to the ear of the recipient(s) across the space not on a horizontal plane but as an *arc trajectory* which travels 'up and over'.

Kaidyn (E, M): I found using the yawn resonance exercise particularly helpful. Why? It was really specific because I was instructed to keep my tongue tip forward so that the back of my tongue would not bunch and block my pharynx. I used the feeling of this sound in the exercise to be an anchor to find a marker to bring more pharynx and chest resonance when I went into speaking. It's physical. Sound, vibration is physical. This and rib stretches helped me find and create more space above and below my larynx so that the sound could be stronger and more projected.

EMBODIMENT

Exercises that engage body, breath and voice, for example by releasing the knees, connecting the big toe to the ground, and releasing the jaw, facilitate development of chest resonance.

Rib stretches are important in enabling the intercostal muscles to be free and responsive. This may be useful for transmasculine and non-binary people who are *binding* prior to mastectomy surgery if this is sought.

EXERCISE: Re-visiting rib stretch and swing

This can be done sitting or standing.

- Raise the right arm over the head; use the left hand to feel the right rib cage expansion.

- Take a slow sniff in, hold for a count of three, and then sigh out.

- Lower the arm, and return to an upright position.

- Notice the difference between the stretched and un-stretched side.

- Repeat with the left arm and side.

VOCAL FOLD MASS

Thinning vocal fold mass can be useful in exploring typical transfeminine and non-binary transfeminine voice work. It is usefully applied to telephone speaking context.

EXERCISE: Reviewing vocal fold thinning

- Using a descending pitch slide on 'ah' which has a simultaneous vocal onset, even lightly glotalized, brings vocal fold thinning – think of sweetening the tone. Ensure that there is no blowing air through the folds and the tone is clear. This is important in your lower range pitches with thin folds.

- In conversation-based practice and group work, using 'oh...', 'ah' thinning helps generalize this quality into conversation.

COMBINED SKILLS: INTONING INTO SPEAKING

Intoning into speaking is a composite exercise combining pitch starting, forward resonance, intoning, thin folds, raised ground and finishing confidence. We have found this to be a really excellent multi-layered exercise which focuses many skills in transfeminine and typical voice feminization work. It really offers a very concentrated workout of skills which can be generalized into speech. The starting place becomes the pitch start – this is the fundamental to raising pitch and has to be habituated. This is useful for transfeminine and non-binary speakers seeking typically perceived 'feminine' parameters.

EXERCISE: All in one: intoning into speaking

- Intone at E3 (165Hz), F3 (175Hz), F#3 (185Hz) or G3 (196Hz) /m/→ 1 2 3 4 5.

- Then breathe after 5, and speak '6, 7, 8, 9, 10' – jumping to highest point on '6' (top of speaking voice – not falsetto) then sliding/ stepping down on '7 8 9 10' (where '10' is at the bottom, the full stop, as it were).

- Note that the pitch of '9' and '10' are *lower* than the intoning at the start. If you return to the starting pitch (i.e. if you pitch on '1' and '10' are the same) it will sound like a *sung* rather than a *spoken* phrase.

- Keep 'smile tone' throughout and especially on 9 and 10.

- Keep vocal folds thin through the slide/step '6–10' – especially to the lowest pitches on '9' and '10'. Enjoy inhabiting the finishing pitch – it deliberately challenges and celebrates the narrative of 'dropping down'. This is a naturalistic rise-fall intonation pattern and you are meant to descend ('drop') – embrace it

- You can try clapping on '10' to create a definite, confident ending enabling the rise-fall contour of the whole exercises to arrive at complete resolution and cadence. Repeat without the clap and ensure the same confidence in landing home.

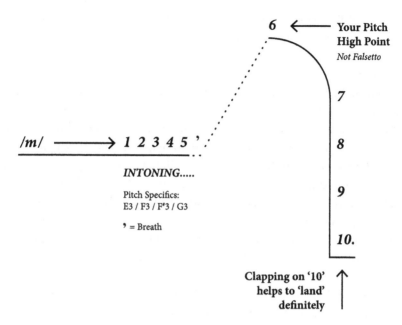

6 ← Your Pitch
High Point
Not Falsetto

7

/m/ ——→ *1 2 3 4 5* ' .

8

INTONING.....

Pitch Specifics:
E3 / F3 / F♯3 / G3

' = Breath

9

10.

Clapping on '10' ↑
helps to 'land'
definitely

INTONING INTO SPEAKING

Combined Skills: Loudness contrasted with intonation

This composite exercise combines resonance, vocal fold thickening, speech quality and prosodic expression through loudness and emphasis contrasting to intonation and range. Use a starting pitch that is easy and comfortable. This is used mostly with transmasculine and non-binary speakers seeking typically perceived 'masculine' parameters and exploring expressiveness, gravitas, and a certain prosodic emphasis.

EXERCISE: All in one: loudness contrast intonation

Choose a sentence, such as 'I am going to see my friend tonight.'

- Speak it with mouth closed noticing chest resonance and vibration on the lips.

- Repeat, exaggerating intonation over loudness. Repeat with the mouth open.

- Repeat, exaggerating loudness over intonation. Repeat with the mouth open.

- It can be helpful to think the sound existing on vertical plane for intonation, and a horizontal plane for loudness – in terms of directional movement.

SINGING

It can be helpful to use solfege 'Do-Re-Mi-Fa-So-La-Ti-Do'. Overall, exploring relationship to speaking, consider voice quality, and use major second, ascents and descents, and scales to major thirds. These very small increments enable clients to negotiate the passaggio – the so-called 'break' – in the voice, which will have shifted on testosterone and vocal fold thickening. Professional singer clients will have singing teachers, with whom we can liaise. Non-professionals, who seek to work with improving singing, can choose songs at a personal pitch comfort, away from Soprano-Alto-Tenor-Bass (SATB) rigidity which is highly musically standardized and typically cisnormative.

Stephen (E, M): So, it took me a while to getting around to exploring my voice after it changed, because the narrative around voice change for transmasculine people is that it's a loss of proficiency, a loss of range and a loss of flexibility – rather than a 'change'. Particularly the older you get, when you transition, the narrative is always that you won't have a strong voice, you might be 'trapped' in a 'small voice' – to the point that people often don't take t because they are singers and they might be worried they are going to fuck up their voice. There's a journey there in realizing actually there are still possibilities, and allowing yourself to explore them.

The physiological changes mean that you lose a bit of stability, certainly early on. And I think a lot of voices pre-t or 'feminine'-sounding speakers tend to place their voices higher, and if transmasculine people continue to place their voice high in either pitch or resonance after voice has changed on t, you lose stability and the voice tends to crack. So transmasculine people need to re-evaluate how you are using your voice in order to start feeling it *as it is*, if that makes sense. So, I can feel my voice is more resonant because I am allowing the muscularity of the core of the voice change to be in my sound, and I am not pulling away from it, or over it. The feeling of change goes with using my voice differently, not just the feeling of the vocal growth on t.

The tricky thing about the adjustment period for transmasculine speakers and particularly singers is the loss of control, because all of your learned technique is dependent on what you have physically, and as that changes, the technique becomes irrelevant. So, for me if I am trying to pitch something high as I used to, I have the muscle memory of that but it doesn't work, to the point that for a good couple of years I had trouble even pitching accurately, and as somebody with a good ear that was really frustrating, because I really could hear it but didn't quite have the technique to fix it because I was trying to fix it the way I would have had before!

So, it's important to consult with singing teachers, and if speech therapists have singing training and skills in this area, offer a gentle exploration of the singing voice and how it relates to speaking.

Kaidyn (E, M): From my professional singing training and performing musical theatre, etc., I know voice is best produced with the right amount of tension – from a relatively relaxed larynx. Speech therapists who are not professional singers don't need to worry. Check with the client's singing teacher. Finding my lower register and re-negotiating access to the top of my voice took a long time and gradual process – it's still happening – and exploring onset, placement, my 'breaks', falsetto, are all helpful if it's within the therapist's skill set. Relate healthy voicing to my speaking range and support. Whatever level the speech therapist is working at, it's important to know there's a kind of grieving process for the voice that has been 'lost', and a discovery process for the voice that's being discovered. It takes time to establish. It was good to be reminded that I have one voice which does many things – the choral singing in group therapy helped for all of us to hear how individual men's singing voices can be.

Fundamentals in vocal coaching

- **Giving feedback:** steer away from evaluative, praised-based language, for example 'good' to being specific about what went well. 'I noticed that…', I heard that…'.

- **Pause and reset:** using the same sentence three times, where first and third attempts match, and where there is a 'drop' or change on the second time, which needs to be 'reset' or picked up. The skill focus is to be conscious of the reset. Increase cognitive load and difficulty with three different consecutive sentences.

- **Spectrum contrast**: this has been called 'negative practice'; we favour 'contrastive practice' as it moves away from binary either-or thinking and experiencing. Formulate the vocal contrast with the phrase 'this, and this' rather than 'not this but this'. It is highly effective in encouraging awareness of new sensations and their generalization.

- **Offer big**: in praxis, offer big so that is can be trimmed down; it is hard to grow something big. 'Overdoing' relaxes into being naturalistic through use.

- **Silent rehearsal**: hearing the pitch start, the voice quality, resonance tone, the whole voice *a split second before one speaks* – in a reflective moment facilitates the way to automatic voice and unconscious competence. Silence is not the absence of sound, but the presence of inner listening where we may attune our mind's ear and recall sound and sense memory (Sontag, 2009).

Lucy (E, M): If I feel my voice has slipped to a place I don't feel comfortable, once the sentence is finished, I can reset in a moment of silence to a starting place that is higher, if I want.

Gwen (E): If you can get your new patients to a point where they are confident enough to practice in their own time, the rest of it carries itself, with feedback and checking in, and becoming more and more independent. The moment I started to be confident to sing in the shower, was the moment that I started to notice the difference that I had started to own my voice. It's my voice.

Jenny-Anne (E): There can be quite a lot of trans people critical of other trans people who try too hard to present in a typical binary way and voice. So it is a complex picture. Be open, transparent and adjust to your client's perspective and follow it to their own particular point of independent development and comfort.

Indigo (E): I would say to speech therapists: recognize that this work is about someone's unique journey and not projecting any kind of assumptions on to people. Some people may just want to feel more confident and congruent with their voice – they may not be taking hormones, because maybe they can't medically or don't want to, it may have a professional impact if they did; some people's voices are going to change through taking hormones and other people's aren't. I am speaking in gender diverse terms here. I have said before that I was petrified in coming to speech therapy that I was going be told that 'men speak this way and women speak that way' and was utterly relieved that this is not in any way a fixed concept or focus of the therapy. It's about working with someone to individuate in terms of their own voice. It's about working with the whole person because it's about connecting beyond just a voice. This is not a 'cut off voice'. It needs to be within the context of a holistic human being. Speech therapists also do not need to feel they have to be miracle workers. People can come to you with expectations that may not be achievable, and it's important to work with someone to process what their fantasises and hopes and dreams are, and when actually they may not be able to fulfil those, and when other journeys may be possible, and what it might feel like for that person to have potentially a sense of loss, not only the joy of the gain.

Gwen (E): We move from individual to group sessions and being authentic – that's the thing. During one of the early group sessions we had some very heart-felt stories about some very personal connections, things people are passionate about, during some of these presentations, things got emotional – there were tears. No one jumped in to save them. The best thing was that they were crying and being themselves in their authentic voice. If we don't allow ourselves to be vulnerable, we are not being honest with ourselves and I think we show strength and invite people in when we do this.

PART II SUMMARY: BEING THE VOCAL COACH

- Trans and cis people perform gender vocally.

- We have one instrument and many voices – code switching.

- A flexible voice is a healthy voice.

- Celebrate yours and your client's voice today as whole and valid.

- Start with highly structured practice of parameters, especially in pitch raising, using masking and rhythmic turn-taking, then move flexibly to handing over the practice and facilitating client independence.

- Relational voice work is the heart of the exploration.

- Demonstrating new and non-habitual vocal parameters for you is essential in sharing risk and discovery.

- Use directional and spatial visual feedback with gestures which illustrate and shape target sound.

- Think beyond binary construct, but don't take it away from anyone who values it.

- Your vulnerability, flexibility and imperfections are your friends.

- Embrace imposter syndrome for the benefit of you and your clients.

- Be mindful of vocal transference and countertransference.

- Minority stress and marginalization may significantly affect your client's ability to participate and practise.

- Confidence emerges from conscious competence.

- Acknowledge the paradox of change: 'you are allowed to change but you don't have to' is the central tenet.

- Spectrum contrast, pause-reset and silent rehearsal build secure skills.

CHAPTER 4

The Social Space

CONTEXTUAL AWARENESS

THIS CHAPTER WILL ASK

What is our experience and understanding of group process and practice?

How do we support progression from individual therapy into voice groups?

How do we combine the roles of facilitator and coach to hold a space of opportunity for practising voice and communication goals in more complex vocal situations?

WHY GROUPS?

McLaren (2016) said that 'We do not stand *before* the social world, we live in the *midst* of it' (p.133). We would be doing a dis-service to many people if we limited therapy to individual sessions. The benefits of group work for trans and non-binary people have been well documented in recent years (Mills, 2015; Mills and Stoneham, 2017; Mills *et al.*, 2017; Pert, 2019; Stoneham, 2015). Follow-up attendance in a group programme is discussed with clients during individual sessions so that, as they develop awareness about using their own voice, they may be considering the benefits of extending knowledge and skills beyond interacting with a clinician. The more diverse group community of learning and support enables exploration of voice within more complex vocal situations. In considering transmasculine voice therapy, Azul (2015) outlines three complex factors within these 'vocal situations' that may be challenging for speakers: presentational (the anatomy and physiology of the speaker/singer's voice and their vocal-communicative behaviours), attributional (the listener's perception and meanings they attribute to the speaker/singer's voice) and normative (the cultural, environmental and heterocisnormative lens through which concepts of gendered voice and vocal function are viewed and experienced).

Any social change encompasses consideration of both self and other people within a range of social contexts, for a range of purposes. We know and experience for ourselves our own 'threat and reward' triggers that govern our social responses, and how anxiety may be heightened by a change in how we behave, even when it is desired or will likely have better outcomes in our interactions with others. In Chapter 1, we highlighted the systemic experience of 'otherness' experienced by trans and non-binary people, and how this may contribute to the dysphoria experienced in relation to gender and specifically to voice. The distress and anxiety expressed by clients often results in, at the very least, filtering, possibly self-silencing, and even avoiding social communication altogether in some contexts. Most importantly, but not exclusively, groups offer:

- a safe space to explore voice more freely

- group coaching of vocal skills for shared learning and feedback

- shared exploration of the anxiety inherent in some social situations

- shared acceptance of vulnerability and exploring qualities such as honesty, presence and resilience

- a fun and a playful approach to voice and communication

- practice in transferring preferred aspects of voice into interaction with others for a range of purposes (for example on the telephone, projection, assertiveness).

BUILDING EMOTIONAL INTELLIGENCE IN GROUPS

In group exploration of self in the context of interactions with others, emotional intelligence (EI) can be a relatively simple and useful framework that is used, for example, in education, business and leadership contexts.

		SELF	OTHER
RECOGNIZE (Mindfulness)		**SELF-AWARENESS** Acknowledgement of fear around listener reactions to: - lack of congruence - use of 'new' unfamiliar voice Acknowledgement of vulnerability Awareness of triggers for anxiety, avoidance 'self-silencing' Awareness of assumptions about self and others in relation to voice that act as 'filters' Validation of thoughts, feelings for self-identity	**EMPATHY** Understanding of how focus on own journey can interfere with: - active listening - perceptions of others - ability to empathize Recognition of current skills in recognizing others' responses and emotions – for example, may use fewer questions and learn less information about others that will build relationships
REGULATE (Empowerment)		**ADAPTING** Integrating emotion into action Using verbal and nonverbal behaviours to minimize the stress triggers Changing beliefs, positive thinking and resilience Productively channelling emotions, for example: - remaining calm - honest disclosure	**SOCIAL SKILLS** Choosing appropriate responses for the situation, for example: - building relationships - collaborating - managing conflict Taking into account others' emotions or tension without being controlled by it

THE FOUR DIMENSIONS OF EMOTIONAL INTELLIGENCE

The model can help in normalizing the interplay of internal thoughts and feelings, and how constructive use of these, together with empathic understanding of others, can be used in managing emotions and adapting behavioural responses to people, situations and events. Consideration of all four elements of EI means being present and using behaviours more creatively in different contexts (Ochsner and Gross, 2004), which in turn results in more effective outcomes. Drawing on a cognitive behavioural approach, more conscious recognition of emotions, thoughts and behaviours provides evidence for understanding their influence in complex lived situations and a rationale for learning flexibility in responding effectively in the moment (Slaski and Cartwright, 2003).

This requires the ability to switch rapidly from focusing in, through developing self-awareness, and focusing out, through developing empathy, in order to regulate behaviours as part of social skills. Through self-awareness we become better able to navigate stress-inducing experiences and manage the fight-flight-freeze-faint fear responses that can act as a filter and compromise social interactions. Daniel Goleman (2009) stated that 'emotional intelligence requires being able to pilot through the emotional currents always at play rather than being pulled under by them'. This opens up a more creative space for using empathic listening to take account of both our own and others' needs within an interaction. Using social skills more consciously and purposefully helps us to build relationships that are *value-based*, and therefore more authentic, in a wider range of social roles we adopt.

> **PAUSE FOR REFLECTION:**
> A quick self-assessment of EI can be found at:
> www.mindtools.com/pages/article/ei-quiz.htm

BUILDING RESILIENCE IN GROUPS

Presenting in group sessions is ideal for building resilience to the psychological and physical threats that can trigger stress responses on a daily basis and compromise vocal and communicative performance. Participants can acknowledge the shared impact of these on physiological responses, such as heart rate, sweating or reddening, as well as on the vocal mechanism itself, even to the point of being 'speechless' or 'struck dumb'.

Jenny (E): When you first said, 'You'll get more out of the group', I couldn't see it. But we're all in the same boat, 'locked' in the same room, there to help each other, I'm not on my own. Everyone was nervous but I was the first one out of that chair with my shoes. When you said, 'Who is going to stand up and do their speech?' heads went down, but I got up. The more you worry about it the less you do it. I came away a better person from it. I bounced off everyone – listening to their voices and trying, watching what others were doing. I was trying to build myself up and do the same.

As voice clinicians, we prepare people to act free of any doubt through encouragement to try something out, to suspend judgement and to risk failing.

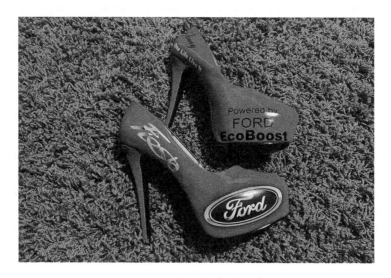

Jenny's ability to take risks in being present and in sharing a personal story about her red shoes was palpable. Trying out pause helped her both *focus in* on managing her internal state and *focus out* on the audience in conveying her intention.

Jenny's red shoes have become a symbol, much like Dorothy's ruby slippers in the *Wizard of Oz*, of finding the courage to change. Lady Gaga owns one of the original pairs of red shoes made for the film and, on revealing that she was bullied in school, said, 'When you don't feel like Dorothy today, maybe you feel like someone on the chorus or the Scarecrow…just know you will have opportunities in your real life to change things and maybe someone, somebody will hand you a pair of ruby slippers.'[1]

Many people will describe this courage as 'being more confident': in reality, the taking of action in a difficult situation results in *feeling* more confident to act in a similar way again. Kay and Shipman (2014)

---

1   See www.thelist.com/34367/things-you-didnt-know-about-dorothys-ruby-slippers

talk about the volitional aspect of developing confidence as 'the purity of action produced by a mind free of doubt' (p.3).

Erin (E): Confidence can be like a self-fulfilling loop. If you pretend you're confident, you 'trick' yourself into it, you naturally become more confident. So, don't think too hard about it! No one's paying as much attention to your voice as you are. Just fake it 'til you make it! You know a lot more about your voice than anyone else does. Confidence comes from knowing what you are doing, practising it so you get really good at it so you don't have to think about it so much, and you can rely on it.

The beginnings of personal resilience require nurturing further if the resulting confidence and competence are to be transferred effectively in more complex situations, and the group builds a community that supports this growth: 'One of the most remarkable of all human skills is our ability to flexibly adapt to nearly every imaginable circumstance. This ability arises in part from our capacity to regulate emotions that are endangered by the situations we face' (Ochsner and Gross, 2004, p.2).

WHAT IS PERSONAL RESILIENCE?

The word 'resilience' comes from the Latin *resilire* – to spring back, rebound. Building resilience can help us to predict future risks and 'future-proof' the way we manage challenging experiences. In 2014 The Young Foundation highlighted the link between well-being and resilience and also an important distinction (Mguni, Bacon and Brown). Whilst well-being describes a psychological state at a point in time, resilience is dynamic and takes into account the past and future. By noticing and managing our thoughts and feelings in relation to past and present experiences, we can build more resilient thinking and more effectively manage stress responses that are triggered. Lucy, Poorkavoos and Thompson (2014) identified five resilience capabilities: managing physical energy, understanding perspective, emotional intelligence, connections, and purpose, values and strengths.

Self-awareness and acknowledging internal emotional state is the first step in becoming more resilient, and therefore learning to manage our responses. Brené Brown (2018) tells us that acknowledging how vulnerable we all are in uncertain and sometimes emotionally intense human interactions is the first step to being courageous. Building this level of self-awareness requires being present and creating space for conscious engagement with thoughts and feelings and what is driving behavioural responses.

Developing a new vocal identity and transferring skills into increasingly complex vocal situations requires the resilience to develop perspective and emotional intelligence. For example, repeated experiences of being misgendered on the telephone may have resulted in phone avoidance, anger and aggressive responses. Stress responses triggered by beliefs around speaking on the telephone may increase and in turn have a direct impact on voice. Beliefs become self-fulfilling and cognitive and strengths-based approaches support therapists in inviting clients to reframe negative thoughts, in turn building more resilient thinking and self-efficacy. Martin Seligman (2011) provides a useful framework within which to explore thoughts around a situation that either help or hinder resilient responses known as 'attribution theory'. Seligman's resilience work teaches psychological skills to 'immunize people against learned helplessness, against depression and anxiety, and against giving up after failure: by teaching them to think like optimists' (p.3). Attribution theory explores causal thinking within three dimensions, related in the figure 'Resilience' to when situations did not go well:

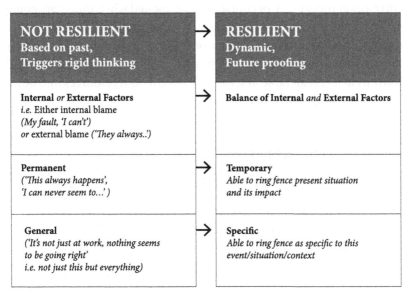

RESILIENCE

- *Internal/external:* If we view the cause of a situation as either wholly internal (down to ourselves) or external (wholly down to others) we may stay in victim mode (the 'I can't' of learned helplessness or a 'them-and-us' blame). Resilient thinking is the 'sweet spot' that balances both internal and external factors.

- *Permanent/temporary:* Rigid thinking may be evident in the use of permanent language such as 'I always', 'no one ever…'. Resilient thinking develops from the ability to ring-fence an unsatisfactory experience as temporary or particular to that situation – which is more difficult when, for example, misgendering due to perceived voice and communication style is experienced repeatedly.

- *General/specific:* Rigid thinking here takes our perception in one situation and generalizes it to others, even seeing that our whole life is a disaster, failure and so on. The ability to be more resilient and consider each situation as specific, as a different experience, may again be more difficult in reality within the wider journey of transitioning, where allowing a true identity to emerge in not only voice but also language, expression, physical appearance and relationships with familiar and unfamiliar others carries expectations.

Attribution theory can, of course, also be applied when things are going well, to enhance positive thinking, self-esteem and self-efficacy rather than attribute success to luck or a one-off. If I accept that success was down to me, I can develop the belief that success can happen again, and learn what is transferable in terms of strengths and resources into other areas of my life. I am future-proofing.

PAUSE FOR REFLECTION:

- Think of a recent work situation when things didn't go well.

- Use the scales below to rate your attribution of the cause, or causes, from 1 (not at all resilient) to 10 (very resilient) on each of the three dimensions:

Internal *or* external   Balance of internal and external

1   10

Permanent	Temporary
1	10
General	Specific
1	10

Listen out for, and gently challenge, clients' language in order to facilitate alternative, more resilient thinking, and highlight resources, for example:

Client: 'I always get stuck with using my pitch when I don't know someone.'

Therapist:

Exceptions: 'Always?...Tell me about a time when you used your preferred pitch with someone you didn't know.'

Affirming: 'In our first appointment, I heard you trying out different voice qualities even though you didn't know me.'

Probing: 'How does that make you feel?' 'How does that impact on the interaction?'

The frameworks discussed in the context of considering group work underpin much of the philosophy and rationale for using applied improvisation outlined in the final section of this chapter. First, we outline group process and a possible structure, and take a look at the art of facilitating groups.

GROUP PROCESS AND A STRUCTURE FOR TRANS VOICE AND COMMUNICATION GROUPS

Group therapy programmes have been reported as effective for trans women and trans men because group cohesion, commonality of experience, shared learning, feedback and witnessing all act as a catalyst for voice and communication change (Mills, 2015; Mills *et al.*, 2017; Mills *et al.*, 2019b; Stoneham, 2015).

Voice exploration groups for trans women, transfeminine and non-binary people

These currently run for five months, at monthly intervals, with a possible social follow-up outside the clinic environment. As the more extensive voice programmes are run regularly, we have explained them in more detail by mapping process and structure onto the following stages of Adair and Benson's action-focused model of group development (Prendiville, 2008):

- forming

- storming

- norming

- performing

- ending.

FORMING

Session 1 is all about creating an environment of safety and a culture of mutual trust within which participants accept the 'high challenge-low risk' nature of opportunities offered. Holding these aims enables facilitators to manage difference: from reticent, nervous or shy responses through to dominant and even disruptive behaviours.

Rebecca (E): There was a trust built up in the group – we're in the same shoes, but we're all different – and we found we had respect enough to be honest and real with each other, though I was nervous at first.

Structure at this stage includes the following:

- Introductory information is given about the purpose and aims of the group and overall structure.

- There are brief activities in which participants are invited to learn names, make introductions and share experiences. Applied improvisation games can help to do this in a playful way, to settle self-consciousness and to include everyone's voices, for example: 'Pre-name-line-up'; 'Ball name games'; 'Name and breakfast'; 'Alliteration name'; and 'Upside-down introductions'(see the

Appendix for these and all other applied improvisation games, listed in the order they appear in this chapter).

- In pairs or triads, participants share best hopes for the group and feedback to the whole.

- Co-constructing ground rules or a contract are agreed on, including some discussion about therapist roles. This is useful here, to surface assumptions and set a culture of universal transformation. A commonly generated contract might include:

  - Confidentiality is to be respected.

  - Mobile phones are to be put away and on silent (unless an agreed reason for being accessible).

  - Be present.

  - Listen to each other and show empathy.

  - Be respectful and support everyone's contributions – recognize each person's pace.

  - Support those who may not be as confident about speaking out in a large group.

  - It's fine to go to the loo.

  - Ask questions if you need.

- A 'boot camp' vocal practice session is used for review of skills, for example hum-pitch, using thinking sounds, intoning into speech, intonation bounces, forward resonance and smile tone. Facilitation fosters discussion around the benefit of listening to others' voice qualities.

- A peer feedback structure is introduced and practised. This might include a 'spot the difference' demonstration of ineffective versus effective (constructive) peer feedback as a catalyst for generating an agreed set of principles, for example:

  - Be specific: 'I noticed that you used a thinking sound to initiate a pitch start'; 'I liked that you used smile tone all the way through that sentence'.

- Separate this from a suggestion: 'Next time you might add pauses to re-set'.

- Focus attention on the other person, rather than talking about your own voice unless invited.

- A couple of applied improvisation (improv) games, such as '1, 2, 3', 'What are you doing?' or 'Yes no' help to reinforce that we are in a *playful* context, and invite a playful approach to voice practice that balances discussion. Play is offered as process rather than the purpose. Improv games also reinforce that the group space will invite exploration of voice within the broader dynamics of social communication: in accepting all responses as 'offers' and that there are no mistakes, a level playing field is created. Experiencing through play, observing others and debrief discussion offer different and rich opportunities to understand our own relationship with voice in social contexts, social anxieties and conflicts over speaking out.

- Key take-aways are shared, including a commitment to action before the next group. Some commonly expressed take-aways after session 1 have included:

  - I can do this more easily than I thought.

  - I'm already feeling more confident in a bigger circle.

  - I've got a sense of where I am amongst my peers – how it's working for everyone not just for me.

  - I'm enjoying the natural conversations – it isn't too forced.

  - It's nice to meet people without worrying about their preconceptions.

  - Everybody's in it together.

Storming

Trust is re-established in each following session. In addition, acceptance of what is in the room and what each individual is bringing with them is encouraged through an initial checking-in. Facilitators' own security in the aims and group process is key to managing group dynamics that emerge, for example resistance, challenge and sabotage.

Session 2 includes the following:

- Time is spent re-establishing names and adding some information in a playful way, for example 'Name and your superpower' in pairs and then back into a whole group for each person to share their partner's information.

- A few moments of guided mindfulness allow everyone to acknowledge what energy they currently have from a) physical, b) emotional and c) mental perspectives. Acknowledging distractions and bringing focus to body, breath and voice encourages acceptance and working with what *is:* a letting go of perfectionism, or a courage to risk more. Mindful breath and body work facilitates individual presence, and fosters a sense of belonging and equal status.

- 'Small victories' and 'sparkling moments' that have been noticed in the time in-between are shared.

- A game to let go and free voice is played: 'President-bodyguard' can elicit feelings and skills around focussing in and focusing out to achieve mutual goals and links to discussion of the components of emotional intelligence. Applied improv games such as this are built in to personalize the group discussion, free the voice and explore the interplay between dynamics: verbal and nonverbal skills, speaker and listener, rehearsal and spontaneity.

- There is a 'boot camp' vocal practice session with self- and peer-feedback. Imagining an ideal voice and silent rehearsal for initiating pitch and voice quality is introduced. This is an opportunity for participants to recognize that we can imagine new voice qualities, and sense what is then happening in that moment of preparing to use it. Guided repetition of this facilitates taking more time and having more choice in how new vocal skills are initiated, and can move participants on from initial hum-pitch and explicit use of thinking sounds.

Facilitation fosters development of critical and intellectual feedback skills, helping participants to both own feedback and focus on specific behaviours. Participants are encouraged to both ask for and provide an individually helpful and appropriate level of challenge as the group progresses. Take-aways have included that it is good to have feedback from people 'in the same shoes as me' and that it is helpful to share reflections on one's own voice first as it gives people a starting point.

Leah (E): The most useful thing is when people reflect on what they've just done. Like 'I was worried about this' and 'I was worried about that' and 'I thought I did this' and 'I thought I did that', and then someone says 'Here's what I saw or heard you do' and it draws attention to what you're probably like in that situation. Does that make sense? I found that really useful.

- Practice is given in using voice on the telephone. We use a short formulaic telephone 'script' to explore strategies such as:

  - recruiting upright posture and facial expression, especially for smile tone

  - using initial and final brightness and bounce

  - rehearsing greeting and ending phrases

  - chunking sentences to take a pause and re-set

  - clarity and assertiveness using 'I' messages

  - holding energy throughout words (see Mills and Stoneham, 2017).

Having elicited the structure, short phone calls are role-played in pairs or triads, with chairs back to back, for honing self and peer feedback on what is working best and what could be changed or used more.

Playing with these strategies in dialogue could include these games:

- 'Telephone Chinese whispers' is a barrier game to manage performance anxiety and self-consciousness as before.

- 'Present in my pocket' is good rehearsal for playing with the bounce in intonation, using thin fold voice quality and managing the potential for self-consciousness when trying additional brightness on the telephone.

- 'Hot telephone': after playing the above games participants are divided into Group A and Group B, in two separate rooms, with telephone access and a facilitator in each. Short, focused everyday calls are made and received to give everyone the opportunity to both practise skills, and to receive feedback from those in the other room hearing their voice through a telephone loudspeaker. (*Some participants may not feel able to make or receive calls at this stage and time in Session 3 gives further opportunity to practise.)

- Key take-aways are shared, including a commitment to action before the next group. Some commonly expressed take-aways after Session 2 have included more self- awareness and confidence of being in a position to know one's own voice the best and what sound is being aimed for.

- Commitment to action includes an invitation to record, or re-record, voicemail messages using strategies that have been found to be most helpful.

Norming

A culture is being mutually established in which all participants including facilitators are encouraged to:

- settle into the group with present energy (see above)

- warm up and practise vocal skills

- give and receive feedback

- explore voice in more complex contexts, including learning from both more artificial exercises and more naturalistic conversation

- learn about themselves and others through facilitated and spontaneous discussion

- state key learnings and take-aways

- have fun!

The culture is more robustly developed through facilitators including themselves within the group process. Participants develop more independence and self-esteem and use their own resources to help others:

Sophie T(E): Teaching is always a good way to learn. If you're trying to explain to somebody else what you see they're doing, you're having to explain it yourself so that you can explain it to them – which means that you've got to understand it. You've got to recognize it, and put it in terms that make sense when you're saying it back.

Session 3 includes the generic structure which is becoming a more familiar way to start each group:

- Small victories are shared.

- There is a 3-minute guided breathing space in which everyone can check in with head, heart and physical energy.

- A short game to free voice and communication is played:

  - 'Positive negative' dialogue highlights the emotion carried by tone of voice and facial expression, and the potential impact of this on the listener.

  - Other improv games such as 'Story one-word-at-a-time' combine cognitive and emotional demands, and require a letting go to accept spontaneous responses.

- There are vocal boot camp exercises and peer feedback:

  - Everyone is invited to contribute to favourite voice warm-ups and tips for maintaining skills.

  - Voice onsets are introduced to highlight differences between breathy, speech and smooth voice qualities and enable exploration in order to both make preferred choices and receive listener feedback.

- Projection: difficulties with projecting voice are shared (often including a perception that projecting voice means reverting to habituated deeper pitch) and contexts where projection may be useful are considered.

- 'Twang' voice quality is introduced and practised contrastively using, for example, duck quacks, miaows, witches cackles, and then in calling out names, greetings, short instructions across a distance.

- Exploring assertiveness versus anger highlights the difference in using personal power rather than anger, and how this may be expressed through warmth and clarity in voice.

- *'Hot telephone' is continued if there are group members who wish to practise in this session.

- Projection and assertiveness are practised through role-play of more complex situations, for example ordering drinks in a bar. Those with mobile phones play music loudly to ensure that there is plenty of background noise, and participants take turns at being bar staff, with customers having to order across others standing at the bar.

- Commitment to action before Session 4 includes the invitation to prepare a short (of 3 or 4 minutes) presentation to the group. This can be read, spoken with or without prompts and on any topic.

As participants themselves become involved in facilitating achievements, new client-led norms are formed that help to minimize the impact of status and the 'expertise' of the facilitators.

Sophie T (E): Sometimes, all it takes is a slightly different point of view, and then all of a sudden you get it! All it takes is for one or another of us to explain something in their way and all of a sudden it made sense where previously it didn't, or it clicks into a situation that it didn't previously. And that's really, you know, really essentially for people who might struggle to understand will understand much better and hopefully it will sink home. So, different styles, different views.

PERFORMING

As part of maintaining this development, participants come to value the human relationships beyond therapist-client, and to celebrate achievements the group is making. Confident behaviours are seen in both individual and group interactions

Session 4 continues to include the regular aspects within the group structure outlined above, with more emphasis on peer feedback in exercises.

Luna (E): Outside this group people are not tuning in in the same way. My partner might say 'Oh you're sounding fine!' Feedback from this group has been specific – what I am and am not doing. That feedback is very constructive. Sitting here listening to each other. Learning how to critique properly. It makes a whole lot of difference because outside of this group feedback is either your voice is 'deep' or it its 'high' – there's no in-between.

- Small victories are shared.

- A few moments of guided mindfulness are shared.

- Games at this stage aim to build confidence in sharing information and responding spontaneously, and to manage emotions such as fear of 'getting it wrong' and other negative listener perceptions. A good example is 'Takes me to the time that...'.

- Vocal boot camp: pause and re-set practice in more complex dialogues is particularly useful for maintaining control in the presentations made later in this session.

- Preparation for vocal performance through the group presentations includes discussion around strategies for presenting with impact in the three key areas of purpose, presence and passion (Goyder, 2014):

  - *Purpose*: this is about intention and clarity of message.

  - *Presence*: this involves awareness of Rodenburg's (2009; 2017) three circles of energy, including demonstration and discussion of their impact in interactions. Brown's (2018) work on accepting vulnerability is important here as are strategies to manage performance anxiety.

    An improv game such as 'Waiting room' may be useful if there is time, and should be played with presence when connecting with others in a group, for example through physical anchoring to 'take the space', pausing, holding eye contact, using warmth and smile in vocal tone and delivering a clear message.

  - *Passion*: A 'speaking circles' (Glickstein, 1998) exercise can be used if time allows.

- Although some group members will not need or choose to present in their everyday contexts, our experience is that managing performance anxiety and focussing out on listeners builds transferable skills. Recent topics to present have ranged from a hobby or passion (see Red Shoes above!), an aspect of transition, work role and an aspect of a PhD.

Feedback on the impact of the presentation and voice dynamics is very affirming, and conversations with participants at later stages suggests that the individual confidence generated is palpable and long-lasting.

Luna (E): Standing up without any props wasn't comfortable. It's something I am not comfortable doing, but that's something I am here to do – I'm not here to be comfortable. I mean I am literally here and I'm comfortable because of the support, but like I'm not here to do things that make me comfortable because I'm not going to learn otherwise. My lack of comfort pushes me to the edge, and the only way I'm going to progress is by staying on that edge!

Daniella (E): I think the confidence of everyone here has grown. The first day we all met to now, it's gone from – one to ten for most people. Would that have happened anyway? Just coming and being part of the group for five months or is there something about the activities being specific to voice? They've sort of made progress quicker. Because we meet only once a month the activities have sort of in a way been like a microphone, allowing things to be faster.

ENDING

As with any group, facilitators need to manage feelings of anxiety and loss that mark the ending of the programme and to celebrate both achievements so far, and new beginnings anticipated.

Session 5 involves the explicit revisiting of earlier group sessions to reinforce the balance of task and process, commitment to change and interrelatedness of members.

The generic structure has become routine:

- Small victories are evident in the detail and language used, and have become more valued through open sharing and witnessing. Confidence to take action is described.

- A few moments of guided mindfulness are shared.

- Games build further confidence in sharing information and responding spontaneously, and to manage emotions. 'The oracle' is a great improv game here, to encourage confidence in being spontaneous, collaborative and supportive, and to reinforce group knowledge about vocal dynamics.

- Vocal boot camp: pause and re-set practice in more complex dialogues is particularly useful for maintaining control in the presentations made later in this session.

Time is given for both formally and informally ending the group sessions:

- Quiet reflection is prompted through re-visiting self-perception questionnaires and vocal journeys and considering change.

- Triads take reflection into sharing of vocal narratives, 'sparkling moments' and strategies to manage challenges in the future.

- Group members often set up mutual support through WhatsApp, phone calls and face-to-face meetings, if they haven't already been using these channels.

- There is a celebration of learning and achievement.

- Some games can be helpful in this final session:

  - 'Wisdom chair' can be part of a final trouble-shooting session in which any member of the circle can raise a query or concern, and someone decides to sit in the 'wisdom chair' and allow an answer to emerge. We ask everyone to avoid waiting until they think they have an answer before taking the wisdom chair, to reinforce the trust that resources *will* emerge spontaneously and will add value to final sharing of group strengths and support.

  - In 'Hot seat' an individual becomes the focus of constructive feedback from other group members for about 3 minutes. The group forms a circle and a facilitator scribes the oral comments. Anyone who does not wish to voice feedback or did not have the opportunity writes brief comments on a piece of paper. All written comments are stapled to a certificate of achievement for each participant. (Note that the facilitator may need to support and re-frame in this activity.) In both of these, facilitators are part of the feedback and aim to make brief comments last to add value to what has already been said.

- *A pub visit* at the end of Session 5 has become part of the celebration of achievement, reinforcing skills and social confidence. This is a great way to free the ending of the sessions in a more formal space, and for everyone to be seen as human beings. Social skills and conversations in the group in a more public setting help with acceptance and authenticity, and normalizing group interaction.

- There may be informal discussion about longer-term group support, although groups have often set this up by this stage, as above.

Voice exploration groups for trans men, transmasculine and non-binary people

Two sessions a month apart are offered with follow-up at 6 months, and potentially 1 year. The following programme forms a suggested protocol for transmasculine voice work:

- vocal embodiment – effect of binding on resonance, rib and back stretches, jaw release, centered breathing and grounding

- optimizing breath support especially regarding vocal mass changes on testosterone

- chest and pharyngeal resonance development – chest tapping, low humming, tongue root release and jaw release

- presence and personal impact

- mindfulness and compassion

- role-play and improvisation of everyday speaking situations, for example, telephone speaking and interviewing

- voice projection and muscular articulation development

- assertiveness training

- discussion topics of toxic masculinity, norms, unconscious bias, cost of authenticity, stereotypes, code switching, queer identities, intersectionality

- singing exploration – range, falsetto, breaks, resonance.

James (E): Voice group for trans masc and non-binary people is a really important space to share and find out about what your voice and body can do – whether you have started on it or not, or are not planning to. Something about sharing experiences makes it possible to go further for all of us.

AWARENESS: FACILITATION PROCESS AND PRACTICE

Awareness of our different roles in different therapy contexts is never more evident than when therapists are facilitating social communication groups. Kitson, Harvey and McCormack (1998, p.153) describe facilitation as 'a technique by which one person makes things easier for others'. Good facilitators make it easier to learn by using their knowledge and skills of group process in addition to the task (Rogers, 2010). Preston (2016) emphasizes the importance of both the *principles* of participant-centred enablement and the *processes* of negotiating with participants. She describes facilitating as 'difficult, messy and full of contradictions and, sometimes, uneasy compromises' (p.1). This requires an understanding of the pedagogy of facilitation that values a process of critical awareness and insight in the moment. In social communication settings, this insight enables facilitators to use the right amount of participation and ownership to ease processes of change towards more effective and creative social relationships. Choices made around delivering a particular task are not simply dependent on technical capability but are driven by the values and beliefs of the facilitator, and in this way draw on qualities of being rather than simply practical skills.

Carys (SLT): Group facilitation is potentially quite challenging because it is a more performative space, for both clients and therapist, as it's an arena in many ways. I think sharing explicit learning about coaching voice change in individual sessions and in group process is very needed. The what, people are learning, the how, too. It helps if therapists have had experience of group participation, even group psychotherapy, to really get the subtlety of what can come up in groups, for you as much as for your clients.

Technical facilitator education

Preston (2016) provides some excellent discussion on the importance of being aware of competing agendas, power relations and of whose interests are being served by the work. By exploring this pedagogy in relation to setting up trans and gender diverse voice groups, we are better placed as facilitators to question whether we are maintaining a neutral stance or whether a particular exercise is pushing a dominant idea or unconscious bias. Applying this pedagogy reinforces the skills of adaptability and responsiveness that enable changes in the moment. This requires that we embrace the risk and vulnerability to accept being in a place of uncertainty with the participants within this complex social context. The whole process demands that, as facilitators, we are resilient enough to manage this uncertainty, however much we have prepared tasks, and to free ourselves from fear and performance anxiety in order to have the confidence to be in the moment. The more we are *aware* of therapist-client relationships that suggest fixing, helping or saving, the more we can moderate these as clients progress, to open up a new unknown culture in which participants can explore their own social relationships and motivation for working together. By applying *critical* facilitation, we can avoid binary constructs such as good and bad, novice versus experienced and examine the dilemmas around more specific binary constructs in voice and gender.

In Chapter 2 we introduced the notion of bringing everything into the room. In group facilitation, our presence becomes an integral part of a space that explores feelings of commonality and difference. If we set up a group purely in terms of having a common need to modify voice, or because of a lack of a particular voice quality, we are in danger of missing vital benefits that a new community can offer those in the process of social transition. Thus how we explicitly engage with this in the first group session sets the culture and helps to establish a community in which everyone is invited to explore voice and communication freely.

A heightened awareness of our own presence in the group enables awareness of different ways of speaking, moving, feeling and behaving. By reading ourselves in this context, we are more equipped to nurture the sharing of previously unexplored thoughts and feelings around voice and social communication; to open up discussion around the pros and cons of considering stereotypical behaviours; and to support desired change.

Thomas (2008) highlighted both intentional and person-centred qualities of facilitators as important within facilitator education approaches (see the figure) and the link to facilitators being fully present and mindful of what makes us who we are, for example feelings, thoughts and memories. Preston (2016) highlights that if group learning outcomes are not met, we may perceive this as a 'failure' equated with incompetent facilitation and delivery techniques, or even participant behaviours. This may result in searching for more *structure* and *techniques* to provide certainty and confidence in therapy practice. If we are constantly striving to have a deeper understanding of the challenges facing our clients, it becomes more evident that 'it's what's between the techniques that is more important' (Thomas, 2008, p.8). By the therapist maintaining a more active and less procedural role, participants themselves can be better enabled to become peer facilitators.

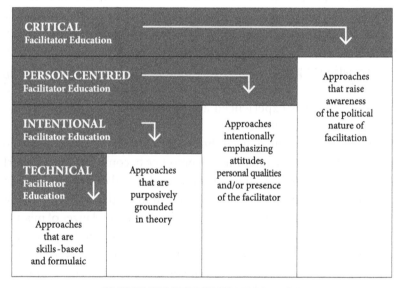

FACILITATOR EDUCATION APPROACHES

Sophie R (E): Hearing the feedback from the group, especially for someone like myself – I'm my own worst enemy with a lot of these things – I'll go away from here and think, 'God, I really sounded crap at that' or 'I did really badly at that.' But having the group say, 'You did well there – it's worked!' that means a lot. Hearing it from yourself is one thing, but hearing it from people who are going through exactly the same does give you that extra comfort and confidence.

Mindful facilitation underpins a focus on physical energy that Preston (2016) says can 'infect the participants in a very positive way' (p.50). This can also help to bring a deeper understanding of the role of physical energy and conscious focus in more complex contextual voice work.

Prendiville (2008) outlines facilitator styles that focus on process and emphasize inclusion and participation:

- *interpretive*: links to empathic paraphrasing to help a participant to find the words

- *cathartic*: encourages participants through modelling the expression of feelings and emotions

- *evaluative:* provides value statements in relation to behaviours

- *sharing:* emphasizes collaborative sharing of feelings about experiencing

- *directive:* keeps the group on track to meet goals and uses reflection, for example, 'Can we just stay with X for a few moments...?'.

As an alternative, Preston's facilitator roles are a useful framework for supporting flexibility and adaptation to group situations, and each one is considered below in relation to trans voice and communication group process:

1 THE DELIBERATE OPPOSER OF THE COMMON VIEW IN ORDER TO GIVE FEEDBACK AND AID CLARITY OF THOUGHT
Facilitators can challenge stereotypes that might foster more rigid thinking and frame client expectations. Whilst stereotypes are undoubtedly a useful inclusion in discussion, they play to binary constructs of voice and communication and may constrain experimentation with behaviours in order to find a comfortable and authentic fit. Facilitators can present important information that values individual style and voice qualities, and reinforces the importance of voice within overall communication dynamics and expression of identity as a whole.

2 THE NARRATOR WHO HELPS TO SET MOOD AND REGISTER OF EVENTS
Group tasks will include 'checking in', for example a mindful space to acknowledge thoughts, emotional and physical states that are

present for each member, including facilitators. Setting an atmosphere of positive commitment and active participation is balanced with acceptance of the energy and focus that people have on the day. Sharing this, for example whether there are distractions that might impact on commitment to the group and activities, can help participants to 'let go' and enter a supportive community with more openness and compassion. Mindful facilitation and solution-focused approaches are important in acknowledging what is in the room, and what resources participants have been able to draw on since the last individual or group session. In this way, 'small victories' or 'stories of achievement' can be celebrated by the group. Facilitators can help to reinforce secondary gains: that is resources that have helped a participant to cope with challenging experiences that are shared.

Within a session, the facilitator's own use of flexible and playful changes in voice and emotional tone, communication behaviours, energy and status set the scene for more playfulness within the group as a whole.

Erin (E): I think a lot of people struggle with phones like being an anxious thing. And that exercise was so funny – it's like having a good experience while talking on the phone. I think that's quite a big psychological thing, a positive experience.

3 THE POSITIVE WITHDRAWER WHO 'LETS THEM GET ON WITH IT'

Using applied improv in particular fosters a process of 'letting go'. The holding of a safe group space, and of the overall structure of a session and its exercises, is crucial in allowing facilitators to engage with their own process of 'letting go'. Stepping back from the place of expert to enable more risk and freedom to respond spontaneously in turn enables participants to 'let go' themselves and embrace being at the edge of their comfort zone. New, less comfortable behaviours can be explored, including transfer of voice skills, authenticity and resilience in social situations. Experimenting with empathy and presence, in particular 'the power of the pause', can bring more emotional intelligence to developing both vocal skills and effective strategies to manage difficult situations, for example being misgendered on the phone.

As participants learn to trust this freedom within structure, facilitators can build in more group independence and autonomy within, for example, peer feedback and support, participants leading vocal warm-ups, and managing more inclusion of quieter members. It is important to include here the 'letting go' of too much facilitator talk. Facilitators who are present and aware are more able to monitor when their intervention may be a result of performance anxiety, the need for a particular outcome or responsibility for a perceived 'failure'. Prendiville (2008) cautions facilitators to be mindful of projection, when what is happening internally may be confused and taken as what is happening for group members.

Adopting a 'less is more' debrief style helps to ensure a solution-focused approach where questions are more usefully focused on self-awareness, sharing of thoughts and feelings, and a *curiosity* about behaviours linked to these. Individuals are more enabled to understand and develop their own resources and to grow a positive group culture that highlights transferable knowledge and skills into the messiness of everyday life.

4 THE SUPPORTER OF IDEAS, AS A GROUP MEMBER

Person-centred facilitation that values individual contributions is the bread and butter of therapeutic group work and needs no further exploration here. It is worth stating, however, that in addition to role-modelling the valuing of all participants, there is something much more powerful in listening to facilitators who accept contributions, even stay longer with them, and then add something (for example, to provide clarity, the potential for greater insight, encourage others' contributions) than a style that reflects back and simply re-frames what has already been offered. Recognizing habituated patterns such as the latter enables us to work with our own self-limiting responses as helpers, and is part of the process of becoming more useful to the group in terms of valuing community and reducing power differentials. In the next section, we highlight the bedrock of applied improv which lies in the simplicity of an 'accept and add' philosophy (Jackson, 2015).

5 THE 'DOGSBODY' WHO DISCOVERS MATERIALS AND AIDS

This perhaps gives a harsh, negative label to what can be an extremely helpful role in running the voice groups. However, when a facilitator is pulled into doing rather than being, over-reliance on structure and technique can provide certainty and confidence in practice. The danger is that this may sacrifice more creative and productive group work that can emerge through letting go and being more responsive to experiencing.

6 THE REFLECTOR WHO IS USED TO ASSESSING THEIR STATEMENTS

Explicit use of Schön's (1987) reflection-in-action – being present to experiencing – role-models the benefit for bringing online reflection and analysis to behaviours. Facilitators can be present with, and then foreground, the feelings and memories that practice allows us to access, rather than intellectual instruction, reinforcing how this supports change and ongoing adaptation of voice and communication behaviours.

7 THE ARBITER IN ARGUMENTS

This perhaps resonates most with the therapist and practitioner as helper, promoting a cultural norm of listening and empathy, and desire to problem-solve. Does this drive pull us into rescuing too quickly? How can we better allow 'healthy' conflict as part of social interaction? Within the complexity of trans voice group work, it is sometimes important to surface and sit with conflict, to name it and allow the group to manage it, as part of managing difference, acceptance of complex lives and competing issues. Being honest and present with arguments can feel uncomfortable, and accepting this enables us to inhibit responses being driven by emotion, by anxiety that we may be upsetting someone. Conflict exists and, as we have explored in depth, it exists in a world that frequently causes shames and distress to trans people. Allowing space for conflicting ideas within the trans and non-binary voice group community serves the purpose of valuing diversity: acceptance of difference; the exploring of stereotyped and binary behaviours; and the exploring of uniqueness within social communication.

8 THE DELIBERATELY OBTUSE FACILITATOR, WHO REQUIRES TO BE INFORMED

Like the supporter of ideas and the reflector, asking for more information can be a way of valuing others' perceptions. The respectful curiosity of a solution-focused approach is useful here: 'I was interested when you mentioned X. I'm not sure how that impacts on voice?' 'What might that mean in the call centre, when daily targets for calls have to be met?'

AUTHOR DIALOGUE: CONCLUDING THOUGHTS ON FEEDBACK AND COACHING IN VOICE GROUP WORK

It takes some therapeutic confidence in group process to give online voice coaching which is being witnessed by the whole group, without making the one being coached feel singled out, but rather, supported. To be able to say mid flow 'Okay great, now try that again and focus on this' can be powerful and thicken the vocal narrative not just for the individual but for the whole group. We include a dialogue below as an illustration of our ongoing struggle with the delicate balancing of roles:

Gillie (G); Matthew (M).

G: Playing devil's advocate, when we invite someone to have another go in the vocal boot camp, and there is little audible change on the second attempt, we have to be careful about the feedback. Using generic praise like 'Great' is not specific, and has the potential to leave group members wondering what we were hearing that they may not. What is the praise for? We are encouraging the 'doing again differently', so in the group we might acknowledge the courage this takes. One way might be to give feedback then coach before a second try, such as 'Hold X in mind when you are trying to achieve Y'. Then give time for other group members to have a go.

M: And maybe handing it to the group to manage as they build more autonomy. There is something in the group about not just the 'either/or' of doing *either* a group activity *or* stopping that person and coaching on the spot. So, what are the shades of grey around group coaching which take account of all those different competencies and confidences?

G: Sometimes that quick win of stopping and saying have another go and try this – that will sometimes be a quick win and people will say 'Oh yes I heard that'. But if it doesn't and somebody is struggling with the target or what that means, what have they achieved by giving it a second go and moving on?

M: So as facilitators we coach, mindful of managing the risk of having another go and feeling a failure in front of others. We balance that with building a community where curiosity and the risk in taking action are valued: having another go and seeing what happens needs to be supported by all group members.

G: And then, after the attempt, opening it up to the group to acknowledge that it's hard to think about a vocal dynamic *and* keep attention on speaking – and that what we are doing is rapid switching of attention.

M: In that way we bring the group into the enquiry and we don't need to give praise or feedback directly for the individual attempt in that moment – that can be an anxiety on our part as facilitators – wanting people to have a positive experience. We're talking about this continuum of directive, detailed coaching to group facilitation to handing it over to the group

G: It's interesting to see what drives us in practice when we are working in the group: 'I really want to coach that person because I can hear that a little more gas under that would make a real difference.'

M: And the challenge is how to get the most out of coaching when there is not a lot of time in the group and someone is struggling with their goal, so that we don't set up pass-fail criteria or leave someone feeling de-motivated.

G: So with a group facilitator hat on, what are the other possibilities in the room? Invite peer coaching. Ask the group for ideas, and what they would be doing to use lifted pitch or smile tone to share responsibility

M: Not rescuing the space, but growing it by handing it over to the group to manage.

G: A situational leadership model is useful here – since we are leading a group structure – the flexibility to move from instructing, to coaching styles that help in developing competence, through into a supporting style that helps in growing confidence, and finally into delegating it to the group as a problem to solve and only stepping back in if it is really helpful.

M: There are times when *I* model a less preferred vocal profile and have the group coach *me* to attain a goal. Inviting the group to be the coach.

G: From observing that, it's a powerful way of bringing the whole group to listen and coach and work with contrastive practice. That is another point – the valuable and healthy opportunity to observe and coach each other as coaches and co-facilitators in a group!

APPLIED IMPROVISATION IN TRANS VOICE AND COMMUNICATION GROUPS

We are including this separate exploration of applied improvisation (improv) because of the growing body of work documenting the benefits of applying theatre improvisation 'to foster the growth and/or development of flexible structures, new mind-sets, and a range of inter- and intrapersonal skills' (Robbins Dudeck and McClure, 2018, p.1).

Applied improvisation is a socio-emotional activity, and trans voice and communication groups are all about creating an environment of safety and a culture of mutual trust within which participants accept the 'high challenge-low risk' nature of opportunities offered. Treder-Wolff (2018) refers to the benefits of experiencing improv as 'a controlled sense of crisis' and there is evidence that the ability to improvise is important in developing our resilience muscle (Coutu, 2002). Holding these aims enables facilitators to manage difference: from reticent, nervous or shy responses through to dominant and even disruptive behaviours.

Although what follows is an introduction to *applying* improv in trans voice and communication group work, the first step to facilitating this work is to learn *through* applied improv. Learning to improvise fosters many useful clinical skills: flexibility, problem-solving, generating alternatives, engaging authentically, acknowledging vulnerability, creativity and resilience to mention a few. There are now many community improv classes and groups where people can learn to flex this muscle.

Above all, the effectiveness of applying improv in any context is all in the debrief and therefore dependent on group facilitation skills. By understanding our own relationship with improvisation, therapists become more confident not only in building games within group work, but also in mining the rich data that can emerge when facilitating the sharing of experiencing and how this might relate to real life.

Improv games provide a low-risk context for people to engage with any perceived threats and stress associated with interacting with others. Complexity and uncertainty in vocal situations can be navigated with more awareness of self and other, and more communicative and social skills, thus drawing on all four dimensions of the emotional intelligence framework outlined earlier in this chapter. Weir (2012) stated that excluded people become *more* sensitive to potential signs of connection, pay more attention to social cues, and tailor subsequent behaviour accordingly. Thus a safe space that provides opportunity to experience social interactions encourages this awareness of social cues and the practice of more effective responses to foster the connections that are desired in real-life contexts. Research into jazz music shows that the same neural processes are at play in the 'give and take' of improvisation as when we engage in spontaneous self-expression – 'like a conversation with a friend' (Paul, 2012).

Furthermore, reflection on experiences stabilizes the cognitive shifts that have occurred and can bring greater understanding of what feels authentic – the aim is not to abandon the self, but to adapt. What enhances our sense of community and significant connection with others? What specific behaviours, and patterns of connection, are useful for this? How does my unique wisdom develop my individual strengths? All this is invaluable for re-writing a positive story on the journey to finding congruent voice and communication. The lessons that are learned create lasting memories.

Gwen (E): There's no script in life! We're not reading a script in life. But the improv and role-play scenarios we did were so useful to deal with the anxiety of having a go. The benefit of kind of performing – not as an actor in a play – but potentially making a fool of myself and just going with what someone is throwing at me, or passing to me – this is a fab life hack, and brilliant, but scary, useful experience. So, I can call on that when I am out of the group and standing in the bus stop in the rain, or being hassled on the tube, or ordering my pizza or espresso, or having an interview on the phone, or just walking through the shopping mall. It's that thing of confidence. I suppose when we try things out and just have a go, we build up our courage reserves and that's what grows confidence. Yes? Improv in the group is all about tolerating the unknown. Having some skills but then just getting out there and using what we have.

Poynton (2013) summarizes applied improvisation as a discipline with three interconnected ideas: Notice more, Let go, Use everything. A well-used single term in applied improvisation is 'everything's an offer'. Consider how these simple definitions resonate with concepts that may be more familiar in traditional therapy approaches, such as presence, being mindful, empathy and acceptance of others. Each of these three ideas can be explored further in relation to voice and communication group work:

Noticing more requires opening the senses to more detail within human interactions that can otherwise be taken for granted. This enables a sharper analytical focus inward on the thoughts and feelings underpinning vocal and communicative behaviours, and a greater awareness of the barriers to success in transferring skills to everyday situations. Skilled facilitation within groups enables individuals to become more active observers of voices and the nuanced behaviours that support change, and to use information to make more effective choices that foster presence and connection.

Letting go requires us to acknowledge the risk involved in changing communication habits: to step into Brené Brown's place of vulnerability (Brown, 2018). The space that is opened up then becomes an experimental laboratory in which participants can learn how different choices in behaviours feel, and the different responses they invite in the moment. Collaboration and co-creation become more important than the control often built as habit by clients to manage fear and defend against the unknown. Loosening this control brings more choices and the potential to flex responses.

Sarah (E): I think it's important to remember that when we have tried our best, when we're talking on the phone or in a social situation, and if something didn't go particularly well, we can remember 'Okay the next time, I will try this'.

What is key here is to facilitate the letting go of habit that carries judgement and to foster the creation of a safe, playful space where no contribution is a bad or boring one. Boundaries are stretched to include the ridiculous, the silly and the more extreme, to encourage more spontaneous choice, enabling participants to both practise a range of vocal and communicative behaviours, and to share their understanding of transferring skills within complex situations. Letting go of assumptions when identity has been so strongly rooted to past experience of incongruence and feelings of dysphoria or distress may be part of the wider exploration within therapy. More specifically, perceived inability to modify voice and communicate effectively may carry strong assumptions and be attributed to causes that prevent resilient thinking. Poynton (2013) points out that the first step to letting go of the rigid hold the past has on our thinking is to acknowledge this 'shadow story' (p.24) for what it is, and that this can only happen when we open up the space to recognize and check what is driving habitual behaviour. Frost and Yarrow's (2016) definition of improvisation emphasizes that 'all human resources' are used 'spontaneously, in response to the immediate stimuli of one's environment, without preconceptions' (p.xv). It is not difficult to consider the importance of this for skill transfer into the messiness of real life situations.

Sophie T (E): 'The Bar' improv was very good. You know we all had to talk over each other. It was so interactive for everyone – at the same time simultaneously to practise the same thing with a 'splash' of actual social situations.

Sophie R (E): Most people wouldn't think voice projection is something you use every day – like a lot of people wouldn't think to practise it as such until you mentioned it and then you think suddenly, 'Do you know what, that's a good idea to do that'. I also found phone role-play – actually on the phone and on loud speaker, so we could all hear each other – it was a very important exercise. Towards the end, I thought 'Really – what is coming next?!' The fact that we did it was something of an achievement – every day I have to use the phone to somebody, a customer or whatever, so having that exercise to go through stuff and actually hear the feedback I found relevant. I'm glad I did it because it has helped further down the line in my actual work. So, that was a really good exercise for me.

Use everything: This includes perceived mistakes with no need to apologize. The concept of using everything means that participants are encouraged to re-frame everything positively, to see opportunity for connection by valuing others' perceptions and interpretations of experiences. When individuals may have been on the receiving end of miscommunication, negative responses and often transphobia, constructing communication situations that represent real life can provide positive and affirming experiences within which to explore empathy and practise different, perhaps more resilient, responses for more effective personal outcomes. Participants have more opportunity to become unstuck by asking for help, to observe others' contributions and their impact, and to learn from sources other than the clinician.

Jackson (2015) takes an applied improvisation framework further in his acronym LIFEPASS: Let go, Inhabit the moment, Freedom within structure, Embrace uncertainty, Play to play, Accept and build, Short turn-taking, Spot successes.

These important dimensions work well when applying psychological frameworks to support voice and communication therapy, and therapists will recognize how some mirror the underlying principles of exploring social communication. Inhabiting the moment, or being more present, supports pace and pause that helps in Poynton's active

'Noticing more' outlined above. Embracing uncertainty normalizes the vulnerability faced by us all and encourages more risk-taking within a safe, supported community.

Justine (E): All the exercises were helpful. I've never been one for putting myself forward in a group. When asking for volunteers I hung on until 'Oh, I'd better do it!' But everybody had a go. If I'd been asked to do games in the one-to-one sessions, I might have been apprehensive but because everyone had a go, the support in the group was there – everybody was there to back you up and give you a gee-up if it didn't work quite so well. Group games gave it often a lighthearted approach which took the nervousness away – allowed you to push yourself on a little bit further.

Repeating initial name games and greetings is important for larger groups, not only for learning names, but also for managing the anxiety, embarrassment and self-consciousness that so often accompanies such real-life experiences.

Throwing a small ball as part of improv games is often used to inject more fun, promote eye contact, encourage pause and preparation, and to allow spontaneous switching of recipient rather than going round in a circle. Acceptance of 'mistakes' in throwing and catching can release tension and promote a lighter, playful atmosphere in addition to normalizing the performance pressure anyone can experience in a particular context to 'get it right'.

As part of voice groups, using a ball can act as a physical anchor for whatever aspect of voice an individual is wanting to focus on:

Stephanie (E): Physically holding something like a real ball – that helps! Having something you can hold and see. You know someone's going to throw it to you and you're about to catch it. And when it's your turn and you have the ball, you have that 30-second breather to think – about your voice and who you are throwing it to. It was good to have it – 'Ah, I've got it now!'

Despite Stephanie's preference for a prop, repeating a game 'as if' there is a physical ball can maintain the anchor of 'pause and prepare'. This keeps energy in the body and encourages focus out towards the recipient, supporting eye contact and voice projection in real-life situations.

Sophie T (E):   It's that connection – you just associate. Obviously when you do sports, martial arts or whatever, you're trying to build up muscle memory. And in this particular instance, you're trying to build a response to a situation where you're actually putting yourself in that situation so that you can remember it more easily at the time.

A point worth mentioning here is that facilitators need to manage anxiety for different individuals, for example those who are neurodifferent may prefer to use a ball if eye contact presents a challenge; those with physical or mobility differences may need a seated game without ball-throwing.

Our understanding of the concepts of play and creativity within applied improvisation validates their efficacy and has contributed to the *confidence* to introduce games and exercises and, more importantly, to debrief them. Skilled debrief is invaluable in helping individuals to reflect on their own experiencing, and to share learnings that maximize the transfer of skills into everyday life. Augusto Boal, the Brazilian founder of Theatre of The Oppressed in the 1950s and 1960s, developed the use of theatre, in particular Forum Theatre, to explore and improvise solutions to problems. This work was designed to support people trying to understand and free themselves from oppression in social situations. Boal used to tell students not to ask what a theatre game was for but rather to ask participants what they got out of it. This can facilitate a range of meanings for the exercise rather than one defined by the facilitator. Our group participants create their own meaning from both their own experience and that observed within the group as a whole. Meanings created from those experiences interact with and build upon previous experiences and beliefs, promoting discovery of how new ways of seeing and being can be explored in daily life.

For example, Gwen articulates the shared learning of the group that emerged in the debrief of 'Present in my pocket':

Gwen (E): And during the improv activity, the skill is to try to deal with what I am being thrown (some group members were nasty [laughs]) – like 'Here's a present – 'Oh thank you, I wasn't expecting a didgeridoo – I have always wanted to learn a wind instrument!' or whatever. It was challenging to do all that, in front of the group, and to remember to keep my voice stuff going. But the more we did it, the easier it got. Having a slightly warped sense of humour definitely helps me!

Games can emphasize the benefit of slowing the pace in order to break the habitual stimulus-response patterns in interaction, instead opening up a space of infinite possibility and seeing what happens. For example, the requirement to mirror a partner's speech in 'President - bodyguard' elicits the benefits of sharper focus on the other person, enhanced facial expression such as smiling, and contrasts experience with everyday habits such as speaking quickly and using less expressive vocal dynamics.

Dee and Daniella provide valuable insights from the applied improvisation games 'Telephone Chinese whispers' and 'The oracle':

Dee (E): I think it's because I envisaged being in that situation at work a lot and I role-played how I was at work, and then I was able to take that back into my daily life, and I realized I could put that into practice outside of here. I wouldn't have realized that without doing that interaction, role-play, the telephone game, with other people – no way.

Daniella (E): It helps because like we were saying about small talk, you've actually got something to do, you've got a subject to talk about, a task, a phone conversation, a call. For someone who's not used to talking or striking up a conversation, it actually helps with that. It helps break the ice, breaks the conversation ice, having a workshop game – whether it's the telephone or 'The oracle', it helps doing those stories of speaking about ourselves.

Dee (E): I think some of the activities, because you're gently pushing and prodding us in new ways to try out and get voice, allow us to play around, explore. Like the improvisation we just did, 'The oracle' – you can see when people are thinking about making a definition or story together at the same time, and it makes you realize how you rely on people and how you are even asking people something

CHAPTER 5

Space

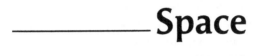

BUILDING COMMUNITIES

If the title of this chapter suggests an empty space, the content is anything but that. It is, instead, an indefinable space of possibility for trans people to continue their vocal journey independently and collectively: where personal resilience and resources continue to grow in a community of support and challenge and where safe spaces are created that benefit both trans and cis people.

It is also a space of possibility for our own growth and creativity as therapists, to continue exploring our own trans awareness and allyship, independently and collectively, and how this grounds and informs our vocal practice.

We invited experts by experience and clinicians to speak about collective spaces of challenge and support where wisdom is shared. The following is an anthology of many lives and stories, including community spaces such as the LGBT Foundation in Manchester: spaces for those who describe diverse communication in addition to voice exploration; spaces documented by couples, families and young people; therapeutic spaces described by clinicians; and political spaces created by all.

Throughout, we invite the reader to engage with these collective spaces and in doing so give this chapter your own heading.

COMMUNITY SPACES
Sean (SLT) talks about the LGBT Foundation, Manchester:

Trans people may have never, or have not often met other trans people to discuss communication, and what that might be like. And I think particularly when people are in the early stages of exploring their identity, they are highly nervous. So, a lot of the clients I see at the LGBT Foundation, we offer them changing facilities, so they are able to wear their version of authentic clothing for the first time – they are in a safe space to be themselves. The LGBT staff are highly trained so they are not going to misgender clients, often staff are trans and non-binary themselves, which gives a strong community link. It's not just a safe space but a relaxing, freeing space.

I have volunteer speech and language therapist students from the University of Manchester assisting me in the voice and communication programme. When the groups start, we might have trans people sitting on one side and cis people sitting on the other, and I say – 'let's mix around and get to know each other!' Many trans people may have stereotypical views of gender performance, and I talk about heteronormativity and that one day I hope we won't be doing this job for trans people. I notice that a lot of trans participants are really surprised that cis people also find gender stereotyping problematic, and performing the voice that they would like to do. So I give an example of myself: I am a gay man and I am out, I have quite over the top nonverbal movements, my resonance may be heard as sometimes more 'feminine', my communication style might be perceived to have 'feminine' characteristics by normative heterosexual men, but I like those things about me, and I am not giving them up, thank you very much! I am very happy in my identity and I would like my clients to feel the same. You [Matthew] have championed your own identity as a gay man, queer, individual, activist, and that's been an inspiring voice in the mix of many speech therapists who deliver this work to people who are also searching to be free of shame and be totally themselves.

A lot of this is about safety. If people have the goal to 'pass' – that terrible term – then they know they are safe. Students find it really useful – we all need to hear from trans people – the horror stories, i.e. how pervasive transphobia is: telephone banking people cutting people off, trans people feeling that they are going to be attacked – genuine fears. The fight to be real. The whole group is an exploration.

The elimination of shame is my deep motivation. A lot of queer people or LGBTQ+ people will have a common experience of that. There's a visceral experience of not being okay from a very young age where society is rejecting, and tries to shame someone into thinking you are not valuable or worthwhile. I dealt with that a long time ago but it does come back and I am a white, middle-class, highly educated leader in my profession, with a lot of privilege – and if I feel like that what on earth must other people without those privileges feel? So, it's about saying to people – you are enough. You are worthy of help and attention. The LGBT Foundation do that brilliantly. People need thinking time with support which is delivered holistically – exercise classes where people can change without feeling awkward – it's a community model. Holism is embedded. Community ownership is enormously helpful in combatting shame: you are part of a community that is strong and vibrant.

It's 50 years since Stonewall! It was *trans women* who did most of the work for that because they were so far away from society's idea of the norm, whatever that is. It's a cultural competence to understand this history because it informs the life experience of most people who are queer in some regard or another. We don't just come out once – we come out constantly. I was working with a trans woman who had what might be typically understood as such a feminine gender expression, including voice, that she would never be misgendered or seen as anything other than normatively female/feminine, and she came as a volunteer, and I was wearing a 'some people are trans, get over it!' t-shirt and she said to me, 'I couldn't wear that t-shirt.' And I asked why, and she said, 'It's my worst nightmare for people to know that I am trans.' And I said, 'I think you still have some work to do which is why you probably volunteered.' Being proud of being trans is something to aim for. And she did end up hanging out with a group on Canal Street and feeling far more connected to her identity.

Sophie R (E) and Scarlett (E) talk about the importance of a social network after the voice group ends:

Sophie R: The whole social aspect outside the voice group is really important because you are practising voice stuff in a real social atmosphere. It is great that our group bonded really well and we formed a WhatsApp group so we could check in with each other in between sessions, and now that the therapy has finished. We can be there for each other, give encouragement, hear about what's going on for people – not just about voice but also about life things. We have social events – going to the pub, having food together. Some of us are confident, some of us are shy, but we support each other! Just great to be there together and hang out, and have the therapists join us for the last session and a social catch up – it makes us feel like actual human beings. The girls, as we call ourselves, talk about voice, dresses, relationships, work, give each other tips – we are kind of doing the things that young girls and teenagers tend to do but we're doing them a bit later in our lives, and that's okay, it's so important to have this support, and that came from the bonds of trusting each other in the group sessions. It's moved on and developed. Our group now nudges you on if you're having difficulties or not feeling your best – we keep growing, and meeting up in public spaces helps us. We are our own leaders, I suppose, and it's lovely to welcome our therapists as visitors, as part of the social times.

Scarlett: We all have to learn to be kind to ourselves in every minute of every day. It's hard but we have to. I am my own worst enemy – the group has been so good for me, and it has value far beyond the voice part – socializing together, it's a community.

Jenny-Anne (E) talks about her spiritual community, and setting up a community house:

I use my voice in all sorts of different ways – on the phone, doing a presentation, leading a service, speaking to a friend. I use my voice in many contexts and would expect the therapist to help in all these aspects. My therapists gave me confidence to use my voice, even perhaps sometimes when it wouldn't meet the expectations of the audience. I sometimes listen to recording when I have given interviews on the radio, for example, and recorded services in church. In church, in particular, I try to raise the power of my voice, even though amplified, so that it reaches people in a physical sense so that it sounds clearer. And I sometimes hear it back as sounding more masculine, but as my pastor said to me once, 'Jenny-Anne never mind the girly voice, project'. And when you listen to accomplished actresses like Judy Dench – cis women of a certain age, they often have a low-pitched voice which is powerful and not girly, and that's appropriate for them. I give myself permission to send out the vibration of my voice. I bring self-acceptance to my sound through the process of speech therapy.

And the community gave me permission to be me. We really want the community to expand in its widest sense and hope that this will be a consequence of this book and other endeavours to bring trans and cis perspectives together in a spirit of genuine mutual respect for difference and commonality.

We all have to learn to be realistic. As clients, we have to understand to distinguish between what you'd like to achieve and how much of that you can realistically achieve. You have to learn that it's okay to be trans. We all have to be realistic. I had been on one or two quite challenging interviews, where people call in to question your validity, and more than one radio interviewer has said to me, well you don't sound very female, and my reaction to that is that well, lots of women have deep voices, and some men have higher voices, they are still the people they are, and we don't have to get in to this thing of only being validated by a privileged or stereotypical standard, but we can just be respected together with everyone else for who we are!

Confidence is developed through interaction with other people. Particularly if you have people who are friendly and supportive.

One of the things that we do is that people who are just starting on their journey are invited to come to stay in our community house because it's a place where they can just be themselves. Then my partner Elen says, 'Come to the supermarket with me'. And people will go off with her, as a social experience of sorts, and local people know us and are generally very accepting. This very nervous person will go with her and when they come back, they're all smiles, and I ask, 'How did it go?' They reply that 'it was a really good experience and the girls on the checkout chatted to me and accepted me'. That engenders real confidence.

Kate Nambiar (E, MD) speaks about supporting community from a medical and lived experience perspective:

The role of 'the community' in healthcare is typically used to collectively describe the patient group that we are caring for. It is less often used to describe a group of people who are not only receiving healthcare but are actively involved in designing, shaping and delivering that service. Unfortunately there is much that needs to be done to improve healthcare for trans people. As a doctor I have heard patients tell me that they have had to face discrimination and lack of knowledge from the people caring for them; and as a trans woman myself I've seen first-hand how inequalities in care can be detrimental to my own health and well-being.

When we started Clinic-T (a sexual and reproductive health clinic for trans people) we wanted to ensure that the trans community would not have to face those inequalities by embedding the notion of *community* within the fabric of the service. It was our patients – trans people who felt that existing sexual health services were not adequate for their needs – who asked for the clinic to be set up. At the time we started in 2012 one other service, cliniQ in London had only just begun to offer the same community-led model of sexual health and well-being services. We worked together with them to implement training for our staff in Brighton and we employed volunteers and staff members (me included) from the trans community to run the service. Over the years, the nature of what we do has changed to meet the evolving needs of our patients. We moved from being a gateway service engaging people with an existing sexual health department, to one where we were providing specialist care over and above what was available in conventional services, and where we were described by our local council as 'an asset to the trans community'. I am very proud of what we have been able to achieve, and there is much more yet to do, but I am certain that we would never have been able to get where we are without being a service that was 'By Us, For Us' – enshrining community at our heart.

DIVERSE COMMUNICATION SPACES

Pippa (E) writes about her stammer:

I had speech therapy for my stammering years ago, but I still often get stuck. Blocks. Repeating. It was really helpful to realize the link between stammering therapy and voice feminization therapy. When I get stuck, block, repeating, I remember the image of trying to pull a door open but not getting my foot out of the way. It won't work! Struggle! Ugh! When I get my foot out of the way and open the door, I get into my flow and out of blocking or pushing or too much tension. My voice feminization started with revision of my stammering therapy and I realized that pitch and tone exercises also get me into that flow too, that humming quality, voice moving, aiming up without pushing, open throat feeling, and that gets me straight into my best feminine voice.

Keeping eye contact, and using flowing, not tense, body language, keeps me connected to other people. Telling stories, in the group, helped me practise feminine voice and stammering together. I didn't pull away into myself. Not avoiding difficult moments helps me actually use my best feminine voice. I have to face being realistic all the time with my stammer, deal with it, get through it. I have to go for what is realistic. I aim for a low traditional feminine pitch, not high or falsetto sort of voice, because that is what is easy for me and sounds natural for me. Getting my message across, using that smiley tone technique and keeping my flow are my priorities. People accept me for being me. I've had positive feedback from friends and colleagues about my voice. Okay, it's a gradual evolution, and that's okay with me.

I am happy to use my current level of feminized voice range without getting screwed up about it. I don't pretend to be a cis female so I avoid copying and therefore I am evolving my own level. I have good and bad days with stammering but the long-term trend is clearly a great deal of fluency and confidence since I had therapy. If I have a bad patch I consciously remind myself not to get hung up on it. It's not important. I use the comparative technique a lot too. Say it like this, then like this. That really simple technique is a real winner for me.

Stammering and voice fem are linked by challenging my avoidance – good to have therapists who can walk the rocky road with me and get me to embrace who I am.

Nicky (SLT) adds:

I am really struck that many trans voice therapists also have experience and skills of working with adults who stammer, and have gained training in a wide range of psychological approaches to help identity shift process, attitudinal change, exploring avoidance, shame, mindfulness, acceptance, gaining presence. I find the COM-B model (Michie, Atkins and West, 2014) helpful as it offers a framework for the capacity, opportunities and motivation.

James (E) and Linda (E) write about being trans and autistic:

James: How has being autistic and having gender dysphoria affected me? I'm a lot more direct. I don't tend to hedge as much. If I say something, I don't skip around the point. I make people uncomfortable, being very honest. It can help me present a little more masculine – guys tend to be more direct. But, as soon as I say something, I overthink it a lot. In my head, I can't take it back. I might regret what I have said. Dealing with the consequences of being direct. I can be blunt, then I ruminate, which leads to anxiety – a sort of post-talking anxiety.

I would recommend when working with patients who have ASD and gender dysphoria to help them understand that change will not happen overnight and make sure clients don't overthink too much – it can hinder the process. Help people examine expectations and then let go of them! Speech therapists know that ASD can present itself in many different ways, and that some individuals may find it really hard to talk in certain situations entirely, so keeping in mind not to push them too extremely in ways they react negatively to – we are more likely to close off quicker and make much slower progress as a result! It was really helpful exploring in a group of trans masc, non-binary, trans men – we explored together.

Linda: My parents noticed I had some communication difficulties and I was diagnosed with ASD at aged four years old in infant school. I proceeded to a specialist ASD school on a part-time basis, and this helped me work towards developing and understanding social and communication skills. In particular, I learned to try to keep calm when speaking and think what I wanted to say. I still have to be conscious about what I say as I can stop part way through sentences. I find some difficulty in interpreting phrases and jokes, and sometimes tone of voice can be confusing. I always knew I was different in other ways. When young, I played with girls and girl role games, if we can call it that. I started transition aged 36 and my gender dysphoria has lifted considerably. Now I am more focused on my ASD again and keeping calm. Over the years, I have learned strategies in difficult social environments, and understanding the expectations of female gender role has been something of a challenge in terms of communication. It is hard for me to initiate one-to-one conversation.

People with ASD who are trying to feminize their voice because they have gender dysphoria need to relax, and not work ourselves up into too much stress. It's hard feeling out of control. But it is not a race, and you can communicate at your own pace and give yourself time. You will achieve more with your voice if you take time and remember to focus on your listener too. It's very worthwhile being part of a voice group. With the voice group I was in, we were all working towards a common goal of feminizing our voices, according to what that meant for individuals, and developing more awareness and confidence in using our new voice pattern in different contexts. This common goal made it easier for me to fit in. It gave me the opportunity to try out my new voice in a challenging but safe social environment, where people were supportive. Receiving direct, constructive feedback on my voice and how it sounded was particularly useful – because I was quite stressed about the tone that was coming out as I couldn't hear it as others do. I also was quite surprised to receive feedback from the group that I expressed myself with a sense of humour and that impacted on the group, making it fun – it endeared me to people.

I would remind speech and language therapists to help your client focus on one thing at a time and get better at it before trying to do multi vocal tasks – where you start the pitch, intonation, tone of voice. Don't forget the basics such as eye contact! Be patient and give me time to respond – I hesitate and being under pressure causes me distress. Visual aids such as drawing voice and intonation pattern were really useful for me as it made the targets really clear about what I was aiming for. Hearing therapists demonstrate voice was very helpful, and to have things broken down into very small steps – raising pitch, doing the smile tone on top of that and moving intonation around and practising it with others.

After therapy now, I still use counting to establish my comfortable feminine pitch – I use this in my day job when testing microphones ('testing 1 2 3') on mobile phones, and I hear it back! Help people find specific strategies and contexts to choose a range of different voices for different settings.

Naz (SLT) and Ioanna (SLT) add their perspectives:

Naz: Concepts around voice are quite abstract, so if we can spend more time making things as clear and specific as possible. It's on a person by person basis. There's such a diversity of gender diversity and gender expression, and there's such an enormous range in neurodiversity. We all have differing skills in social communication and sometimes I get a bit preoccupied with activity – what a person is doing, or their social functioning – but that's mine to own, it's not necessarily the client's concern, and it's not for me to attempt to impose what I find meaningful versus what someone else finds meaningful in terms of what it means to live a full, active and meaningful life. I revisit the means, reasons and opportunities for communication – a useful reminder for all of us.

Ioanna: It's important to be flexible and adaptable in the therapy we offer, and of course speech and language therapists know this. Working with ASD, as many of our clients have this profile, I find it helpful to use visual-based feedback in particular – such as PRAAT – so that clients can understand and match pitch and intonation targets. Clients on the spectrum also tell me that they enjoy and find it useful to engage with the detail of measuring pitch in objective ways. I also find offering situational templates – scripts – really helps clients to cope with social anxiety and prepare themselves for communication in ways that make themselves feel successful.

CHORAL SPACES

Stephen (E, M) describes his work in music and theatre arts:

The impact I see with the choir I lead is comfort level and a sense of community. People feel more free to push themselves if they feel they are amongst friends or in a non-judgemental space, a safe group of people. They feel safe to try singing in a different part and in a different range, where they know they are in a group where other people are doing the same thing – exploring. And/or, they are finding ways to be all right with the voice they currently have. It's a non-auditioned choir where the primary goal is to sing together and enjoy that feeling. We do a long and gentle warm up. We do lots of stepwise motion and small arpeggio patterns because you want to get people to have an intuitive musical literacy as well as small vocal intervals being much easier to manage. Transmasculine people tend to have smallish 'trapped' voices, particularly if they have just transitioned, and taking that time to let go of tension is the biggest technical thing they tend to need. Having a small voice box means they might be more prone to feeling more tension, and if you squeeze it more, it goes to hell! So, learning to release and gently use the voice is crucial – this has a big positive impact on people's perception of their own voice and their ability to use it.

I feel less self-conscious in exploring singing voice than in speaking voice, because it feels more like a technical skill and less like a fundamental identity. And this is where the integration with speech therapy is useful.

A lot of people come to our improv groups because they are shy or socially anxious about public speaking, and they are hoping to gain social skills, for the lack of other descriptors. To an extent it does help with that, but I think it helps people to own their personality and how it is and be more resilient about the value of their own contribution. I do a lot of diversity work with improv and it's really, really valuable for finding what people's gut reaction is and exploring that.

WORK SPACES

Christina (E) describes her work in leadership and business networking:

When I do a professional talk, I ground myself, present myself in this way: I am a make-up of many things – gender fluid, trans woman, pansexual, bisexual, white, middle class. My name is a single word, but there's a whole life in that word and I am a complex person! I have become super confident, and empowered to be myself and being seen in my female gender has given me so many opportunities, and I have become a more balanced human being. I remember going back six years, I would never have opened my front door, my curtains. When I first came out at work, I was absolutely terrified. Take the rubbish bin out at work – scared of rejection, scared of my family or my parents seeing me. It seems ridiculous now. But it was real.

When I meet trans people at networking events, we are all different. And that's the case with people's voices. Let people find their own sense of gendered voice as that is what matters to people. I made very subtle changes to my own, and that's okay. Everyone has a different view about where they want to be with their speech.

In the last four years I have done 75 network events where I have spoken for 20 minutes to audiences from 10 to 200 and more. I won the British LGBT award, and 15 awards for diversity – executive leaders list for inclusive companies. It's a privilege to help people develop trans and diversity awareness and somehow I have found the confidence to be at the forefront of that. Because it matters. I don't take it for granted – I have been into Network Rail, National Grid, atomic weapons, BP, chaired a women in construction event for 1000 people. I put a transfeminine face onto a cisgender male-dominated professional group. My voice is not perfect. But yet I stand in front of so many people in really big contexts. How do I do this? I have accepted that I am trans – it's not all about passing – it's about who you are, who I am. I show that Christina (me) is trans, I am just a regular person that has succeeded. I have children, hobbies, a mortgage, hopes and fears, relationships, and wonderful family. The story of my life? 'Nailed it' and 'into places I would never have dreamed of'.

Nina (E) documents her experience on health professional interview panels:

I am an expert by experience and one of the interview panellists for the London Gender Identity Clinic [GIC]. I have been on panel interviews for all multidisciplinary positions, and I've heard lots of applicants' answers to questions, some thought through and successful and some not! I know from this experience what really adds up to being a trans aware professional – whether you're a psychiatrist, psychologist, speech and language therapist, or nurse, or other medic. I interviewed many prospective speech and language therapists for the SLT service at the London GIC, from developing specialists to advanced practitioners. I was also informed by my own personal experience of having (a few years ago) very in-depth voice therapy.

At interview, I want to discover why you want to come into this field. Because it's about identity and challenging the status quo, redefining what we expect as 'normal'. I want to know that your interest in trans healthcare comes from the heart, that it's not skin deep, not voyeuristic. Is it a tick on your CV? Is it on your bucket list? Is it part of empire building towards private practice? If it feels like that, I am scared, I am worried. Of course, we're all entitled to have a job and go home, switch off, but in this field you have to know where you stand on gender diversity and equality at a personal level, or you might do someone harm unintentionally. This is therapy work, right? So you have keep asking yourself questions, and get down to the nitty gritty. That goes for people starting out and for people who are at the top of the field, and have a professional reputation to 'live up to'.

Be prepared and research around. There are papers, policies, community accounts, professional networks, guide books, support groups, etc. to learn from. You'd be surprised how many people feel they can rock up and wing it. Believe me, it always shows (and it's painful) because your answers will be generalized. Don't do that to yourself (or to me)! Ask specific questions to all your panellists (cis or trans); don't ignore the trans person on the panel. They will have been introduced to you as the expert by experience, so you don't need to be anxious about assuming that I am trans and offending. I want you to tell me your thoughts about transforming and changing voice, including your own. You may be asked to demonstrate a voice quality – be prepared. Why not? It's okay not to have loads of prior experience, draw from your experience honestly, but be thought through.

YOUNG PERSONS' AND FAMILY SPACE

Carys (SLT) and Mary (SLT): We were fortunate with our SLT colleagues to be invited to do share space and work with young people from ages 12 to 20 for 'family workshops' at the gender identity development service. We learned that exploring voice is of particular focus to many young people. Adolescence is already such a challenging time for teenagers regardless of their gender identity, and every young person is going through the process of growing, changing and getting to know themselves, which can be very stressful. These young people are additionally dealing with a high level of media scrutiny, one that is accompanied by a narrative that these young people are ostensibly confused, do not know what they want. What we found is very much the opposite.

We asked the group of young people to share things they liked about their voices, what they knew about how the voice works, and what they might struggle with relating to their voice. Many of the participants shared a sense of joy and freedom relating to doing character voices, impressions and accents. This revealed an already-extant willingness to explore different vocal and communicative parameters without the baggage of managing risk. A recurring theme on the topic of challenges was nervousness and anxiety, and this was a primary concern over meeting gendered expectations of voices as it displaces a sense of autonomy and control.

They expressed a sense of fragility, robustness and possibility with their voices and communication, and we led them through a programme of contrastive and spectrum-based practice: speech supported by breath versus unsupported by breath, high to low pitch, forward to chest resonant speech, communication augmented by eye contact and unaccompanied by eye contact. It was easy to encourage playfulness they already had and the idea that voice and communication can be a broad, colourful palette from which to paint.

Importantly, we had the opportunity to listen to these young people talk about their experiences navigating their identities, and it became exceedingly clear that each of the people in attendance had spent much time and thought in a process of discovery and inquiry, supported by each other and their families, that these young people know exactly who they are, and that they know best.

POLITICAL SPACE

Natasha (E, Psy): Voice is both vibration and it is *political visibility*. We become more compassionate and right-sized beings when we stand together, trans, cis, queer, whoever we are, in our fight for social justice, and when we develop communities of support and sharing which cross all boundaries and barriers.

Skye (E, Psy): I believe a useful framework for understanding the experiences of members of minority or marginalized groups is Community Psychology. Community Psychology highlights the role of politics, economics and other power structures on mental health and, importantly, encourages engaging in action to bring about social change to redress imbalances of power.

I think this is an important perspective to consider when it comes the trans community and the services they want to access. Given that it is overwhelmingly cis people who work in these services and hold the institutional power, we should consider how this might affect the way the services are run. I think people who work in these services should be asking what more could be done to involve the trans community to ensure that their voices are being heard.

Sarah Belinda (E): This year was my first Pride. I have precious memories and photographs of friends, old and brand new, from it. My first Pride! We walked right at the front of the procession – I would not usually put myself forward in that way. It was exhilarating. If the world could always be such an embracing community, wouldn't we all be the better for it?

Mary (SLT): You may think you're able to remain apolitical while doing work in this field but to be able to do it well requires a high level of personal inquiry. I've found for myself that the more inquiry I do the more I see that cis people perform gender just as much as trans people, although it's more culturally invisible when we do it because we get to follow a template. You start seeing the ways that society actually frames masculinity as neutral or the unmarked norm in relation to a feminine other. Julia Serano's work really highlights this. A really telling recent example of this was a school in Lewes in Sussex (UK) that adopted a policy of 'gender neutral' uniforms consisting of trousers and blazers, which does not allow anyone to choose to wear a skirt. The students demonstrated against this policy but the opposition to it has come from mostly young cis women who are unhappy about the sustainability factor and the demand to buy new uniforms, which is a different kind of political issue. For a smaller number of protestors this issue was about the removal of choice. The school said they were adopting the policy in service of trans students but it seems more like they were doing it because some of the young women were wearing their skirts too short, so it's a way of policing behaviour that is specifically feminine. For some young transfeminine people being forced yet again to having to dress in a 'gender neutral' way could induce dysphoria. Blazers and trousers are historically perceived as masculine but we easily accept the 'neutrality' of them. Conversely you wouldn't be able to institute a gender-neutral uniform mandating that all students wear skirts. So, we locate neutral as emanating from the typically masculine. We never read femininity as the norm, we read femininity as a marked other – this is part of what defines patriarchy.

The kind of inquiry I've had to do to try to reveal my unconscious bias has illuminated to me the way I perform gender and what my personal risk is when performing gender, though it is no way comparable to transness. I've actually had to sort of lean into my cis-ness, which is about consciously upholding the binary and the avoidance of what is societally viewed as transgressive. My perspective comes from living in a fat body for which I am often ridiculed or harassed. If I didn't perform a sort of hyper-femininity there'd be some risk that I would be de-gendered in a way that leaves me further open to harassment as all fat bodies seem to be either de-gendered or hyper-gendered and hyper-sexualized. Also, for example, there are some differences between cis gay masculinity and cis straight masculinity and performing masculinity leaves you less open to risk (think of the Grindr phrase 'no fats, no femmes'!). We consciously and unconsciously embrace and uphold the binary through our performance of gender to blend in so that we don't have to go through what most trans people go through in a way. Knowing that we all have to perform gender should give us a sense of solidarity that motivates us to advocate for the trans people in our lives.

Carys (SLT): It's interesting because when I speak about my work outside of work, I am very aware I don't speak for trans people, I am cisgender. But I also want to make people aware that trans people are just like everybody else. I sometimes try to get friends or strangers to consider what makes them 'masculine' or 'feminine', and nudge challenge when I come up against something quite strong. I think most people are open to discussion. A drip, drip effect. There's a lot in western, probably global culture at the moment about intolerance for people who have opposite or different views, and so it's important to challenge in a way that can be strong but keeps discussion possible. I love telling people about my job and I enjoy seeing people's reactions.

Jan (SLT): To speak as ourselves is political act. I worked with someone who recently challenged the notion of 'the ideal' in relation to his speech and talked about how he had moved from his more familiar position of *aspiring to meet the ideal,* to the position of *rejection of the aspirational ideal.* He described vividly coming to the conclusion that 'throwing off the idea of the ideal' and 'embracing imperfection' is the only way to be authentic. This can be challenging to do and involves questioning the values of society, what is seen to be 'normal' and the notion of 'the ideal' communicator. In doing this he discovered that aspiration 'holds you back' and rejection of the ideal 'makes your communication better'.

I see the 'rejection of the aspirational ideal' as an *act of resistance.* This could be a great title for a collection of people's stories of their acts of resistance, and I often find in conversation that there are a great many such acts. It's an act of resistance to be yourself, and not respond to pressures to look or sound a certain way according to a normative ideal. Michael White talks about 'self-surveillance' which is a very common and modern way for us to judge ourselves and each other, often seeing ourselves as 'a failure', 'not measuring up' or somehow 'falling short'. The refusal of this 'normalizing judgement' would be seen in White's terms as a political act. I feel it is helpful to acknowledge with clients that when we speak in exactly the way we want to, we step into our unique sense of being and that is a political act of resistance each and every time we do so.

PARTNER SPACES

We end the book in an unashamedly celebratory way with two interviews with couples. Their collective wisdom, and that of the contributions above, have enriched this book and leave us with much to reflect on as practitioners. The dialogues below speak for themselves and are given in their entirety.

Indigo (E) and Ruthie (P)

Indigo (I) and Ruthie (R) have been partners for 34 years. They heard about each other whilst at different high schools, were told they must meet as they would 'get on' and eventually met a couple of years later! Having been a congregational rabbi, Indigo now works as a chaplain in an NHS chaplaincy-spiritual care team. He is Trans and Non-Binary Rep on the LGBT+ & Friends Staff Network in his Trust. Ruthie spent years working in the city and then as a volunteer counsellor with children with emotional challenges. Now a qualified professional dog groomer, she is passionate about her grooming business. Using female pronouns by choice Ruthie embraces her own non-binary view of gender and together with Indigo they celebrate their Queer identities. They have a wonderful Yorkie called Zusya who enriches their lives and generously dispenses love.

North London.

Matthew (M) interviewer.

I: Speech therapy has been a journey for me both literally and figuratively – because of my past history as a child survivor of sexual abuse. I sat in silence for a number of years. I couldn't articulate what was going on, I didn't have the language, I couldn't find a voice. And so, speech therapy has been quite literally finding my voice. Of course, my voice has changed. I spent a number of years before I went on to testosterone [T] because there were some concerns about medical issues, but then when I went on T and started to notice my voice changing, it was about becoming more congruent with who I felt I was, and am – and achieving a greater integration.

M: Has this impacted on your professional and community life too?

I: Without a doubt, because it was a challenge initially feeling like I was affirming my gender identity but my voice was lagging behind. It didn't feel like my voice was congruent with who I felt I was. I can remember once singing at a particular festival, and feeling the anxiety about what would come out of my mouth. And then feeling more comfortable when this deeper voice with more resonance that I had developed with you came out – feeling more comfortable in myself and in officiating at those life cycle events. Because it's also about *connecting* with people. If you are holding a community as I am, you want to be able to connect with the community in joyous and in sad times, not just to be a voice that's disconnected. And it is also about finding your integrity of voice too.

M: The vibration that you have is healing for you and for people.

I: Yes, like a note in tune and a picture being in focus – you see the picture in greater clarity, with more appreciation and with more wonder. Quite literally finding a voice has meant that I have grown in confidence.

R: Yes, I've just noticed Indigo's whole demeanour, his whole way of asserting himself in the world – I am not saying he was a wilting wallflower before, he's always been a very strong person! But there's this sense of – I am trying to find the word to adequately describe it – there is a sense now of *purposefulness*. And a sense of *gravitas*, if you want, of something that is very real and very able to state his case, his story. This very shy individual is now someone who communicates with chief executives in the organization where he works – which is not something you would have done before, is it?

I: No, it is not!

R: Now there's this sense in you of 'I have something to offer, I have a voice, I have an opinion, I want to share that' – whereas before you were very shy, very reserved, almost apologetic for some of the really wonderful things you had to say!

M: I wonder how this has changed you, Ruthie – the relationship you have with Indigo and his voice now – has that made a difference to you in your voice and in yourself?

R: Gosh, that's an interesting one. I think we've always been an amazing partnership and very lucky to be able to articulate how we feel and quite protective in many ways of each other. Whenever Indigo has had a difficult time in community or some sort of negative attention to do with his situation, whether that's to do with gender or sexuality historically, I have been quite defensive and protective and in many ways have said things and voiced things which perhaps he couldn't. Similarly, when I have gone through really difficult times when I have been put upon – a difficult time in a work environment – he can stand up for me and give me my dignity and my voice by helping what was very difficult for me to express. Indigo is finding his voice also through his writing, which we share. And historically – I am passionate about music – we have always sung together.

I: Always harmonized together.

R So when his voice started changing…

I: Ooh la la!

R: It was a little difficult because we had to work out how we were going to *blend together*. The idea of a choir is an interesting one – we think about the soprano, altos, tenors and basses in some music traditions and these are quite fixed ideas – pretty much the sopranos and altos are expected to be female, and the tenors and bases are male – and this is very binary and non-diverse. Actually, there are many female tenors in the church choir I go to. I have been singing in the choir for a long time and I was keen for Indigo to sing along with me and there was a nervousness about where he might 'fit in'. And it's easier for him to harmonize with me when it's the two of us, but in a choir he's 'I've got to sing on that note, and if I don't it's going to sound funny!'

I: I just want to sing and enjoy!

R: So, I took him along to the choir, and I thought if it's going to be too hard for you to sing or learn a line, I will come and sing tenor with you. Actually, that was quite an assumption on my part that he was going to make it to being a tenor! So, he goes to audition to my singing teacher choir leader who is lovely and she says, 'Sing!' After he gets over his shyness, he sings, and she says, 'That's lovely why aren't you singing for the basses?' And I am, 'Hello?! Ok, wow! You go and sing in the basses, but I don't think that I can join you and get that low!'

[Laughter]

I: And also when my voice first started changing, Ruthie did like my morning Barry White voice!

R: Yes, I *do* like your morning Barry White voice!

M: That happens to me too – my Barry White morning voice lasts a bit longer in the day than it used to as I have got older – at last – ha!

[Laughter]

I: I have been doing some work with the Equality and Diversity Manager at work, who asked if I would do some of the training with her. We have been doing sessions for staff, and I was acutely aware this was helpful coming from chaplaincy-spiritual care because we wanted staff to know what we could offer them in terms of support. But I am also aware that I bring my trans identity and being Trans and Non-Binary Rep in the organization. I feel more confident and am voicing something about myself, and making it permissive for people, if they choose to or are comfortable, to share something of themselves.

R: When Indigo first started working with you, he recorded his voice every day. He has been recording his voice weekly since 2015! There is something really nice about recognizing fluidity and change in the voice, whatever that is. And recognizing this is my voice at this moment in time and this is the story I am telling at this moment in time. It doesn't negate the voice I have had before. It doesn't negate the voice or story I might tell in the future, this is what my voice is right now at this point in time, and I think that is something for everyone.

I: It's a blessing.

Tea, chocolate biscuits, and the interview draws to a close with the gentle tones of Ruthie reading the story 'The Soul Bird'.

Jenny(E) and Barbara (P)

Barbara (B) and Jenny (J) have been partners for 35 years; they have a loving family and supportive social network. Jenny works in student counselling and mental health at City University. Barbara had been a boxer in early life, and went on to be a care home manager for elderly residents: now she enjoys being a housewife with the odd bit of trans awareness training for the Metropolitan Police and City University adult nursing course and is a regular contributor to LBC Radio. They celebrated their marriage conversion, which was captured in the documentary *The Second Train* by Tellyjuice (2018).

Islington, London, ground floor flat garden, Barbara's vegan shepherd's pie.

Matthew (M) interviewer.

M: What's been important in your voice and communication journey as wife and wife that you'd like to offer to speech and language therapists and voice practitioners?

B: At home voice is not so important. But it is socially. I know my voice has changed and it is consistent, at home or out, I can feel I am speaking from up here (indicates cheek bones). But it's been a hard process.

J: I guess I noticed the voice thing before you, Barbara, in a way, because I was aware from the perspective of watching other people watching Barbara when we're out. Barbara is Barbara. She's a very feisty person, and if something pisses her off she is just going to be herself, and herself before voice therapy was what you'd call a 'typical deeper voice' and we could walk through somewhere together and when she used her voice, there would be looks, threats and a fracas. I could see the danger that Barbara was in. It's almost like I wanted to say to Barbara, which is awful as I would never shut anyone up, but it's almost like I wanted to say to her, 'Could you be quiet when we're out because that will be safer for you'. She would never do that and it would be wrong of me to ask her to do that but I wanted to protect her, and I thought how can we best manage these situations?

B: I would be, 'What are you f…g looking at?!' It would fly out of my mouth. But actually, it is deeply upsetting. I had to go home and look in the mirror and think, 'What the hell I am doing wrong? Why did I get into that?'

J: And you weren't doing anything wrong. You were just being you, but of course you had to learn to step back. But it's scary, there are threats on the streets. I would want speech or voice therapists to know that you really do need to have trans awareness training to understand the issues that trans people face in every encounter they have, *in every single scary exchange* – especially early on – to go up to a counter or just step out of the front door. We went out a lot together, didn't we, but you also had to face going out on your own.

B: I had to, and had to jump in at the deep end. I said to myself, if I am going to do this, and make this happen, there's no point messing about. There's no point hiding away in my flat. It was hard and just before I told Jenny, during 2011, I actually tried to destroy myself, not kill myself, but I tried to self-destruct. I tried to destroy myself slowly until our relationship went rock bottom. I became nothing. Non-existent but alive.

J: You'd built up this armour, this toughness from early life, hadn't you, being a boxer, and growing up on the streets of Islington in the 60s and 70s, you had to be tough and get respect – you are tough, but inside there is a sweet, very sensitive soul.

B: Those two things are fighting in me. And when I go into fight or flight situations, my voice reverts, maybe not totally, but I hate myself for it. I have a fearsome voice in me, when it comes to protection.

J: There are society double standards – we expect men to behave in a way and a woman to behave in another way, how they express emotion, and that doesn't even take into account people who don't want to identify as either. It was unbearable to me that Barbara was locked away and ashamed of herself for all those years. I couldn't bear it. That was the *most unbearable* thing. It was a eureka moment finally knowing what she had been going through, but it was so, so hard and upsetting to know that she had been suffering. I wanted to take responsibility for it – you have been in prison for all this time we've been together, you silly bitch, why didn't you say so before?! [laughs and tears]. We could have gone partying in the 80s!

B: We are making up for it now! [Laughs]

J: I also absolutely believe that things happen as they are meant to and, horrible as it is that you had to wait that time, you were ready when you were ready. And as soon as we had the conversation, the eureka moment, I said, 'You have to do this within five years, by the age of 60.' I micromanaged it all and stood by every step of the way.

We're living our life today. Life isn't perfect and it never will be, but I wouldn't have it any other way. This journey has been unbelievable, hasn't it?

B: The obstacles have been huge.

J: You have embraced the obstacles, and our determination to face things together and work through things…we've worked through every one of them haven't we? And our family and friends.

B: Yes, and people have respect for us. We reach out to people. We've made it work because we aren't afraid of telling the truth. Coming back to what I would say to speech and language therapists or voice teachers, I would just look you in the eye, and say quietly: *just listen.* Listen to what I am saying. We won't be able to repeat again, just listen to what I am telling you about the problems I am having with my voice and my self-acceptance with my voice, and maybe you can help me with both. If you jump to your conclusion, you will miss out on my story, and I will stay in the shadows. I am unique. The next person is unique. My experience, some of it, might be useful to the next person, but at every stage you're dealing with an individual and you can learn from me too.

J: Yes, I would say to therapists, try to walk beside the person and see from the perspective of the trans person. It's a very privileged place to be, to walk alongside a trans person – it's not just about their voice, it's about the anxiety of using the voice and sounding different. Don't just do 'bog standard' stuff but be really thoughtful about what you are doing and think about the individual in front of you and how you might best support them together with the support system they have around them. Some will have no support. Barbara has me. I have Barbara. Yes, when Barbara started therapy, I could hear there were changes in her voice but I could also hear a lot of frustration that it wasn't as she wanted it to be. She dug deep in to it, and then she plateaued and then she dug in deep again. It was a journey of trying to be confident with something that didn't feel like her own voice. She had to go through the difficult phase of feeling like she was creating something that was not her true voice. I found that very frustrating – I was thinking, 'You don't need to change your voice, it's people's view out there that needs to change, and I wish you could learn to accept you and love you for being you, and work with that.' But I knew that overall it is too hostile out there to do that, and it was important for her to explore changing her voice.

And Barbara *has* changed her voice, and it sounds like Barbara, and it's honest. It was a privilege for me to be part of that voice change journey because I had to deal with my own frustrations, my own biases, which wasn't easy because it was frustrating. But we managed it because we talked about it and did it together.

B: 40 years ago I looked like Ronnie Kray. Now look at me. Now *listen* to me!

J: We're being more human now!

B: We've taken off our straightjackets!

J: We have a choice. We can, all of us, either keep our minds closed and stay in ignorance, or we can be willing to open up a little bit and accept there are a lot of things we don't understand and let's move towards them a little bit. We don't stop being human beings and we can move beyond rigid categories, gender or otherwise. We look to the younger generation and hope they won't be broken by some of the religious dogma and the old school, Neanderthal thinking, and be able to find themselves and speak up and create more accepting communities.

M: Any final thoughts?

J: Barbara is totally herself – feisty, sensitive, and there's something totally spontaneous about her which I love and hate at the same time! [Laughs] Because I come home, and all of a sudden the room's been moved, and then she's singing – but it's wonderful. We have so much fun. When things are difficult, we hold each other and dance and sing together.

B: We play with our voices *together* – play gender voices, we do our 'Ken and Barbie'. I'm 'Barbie' and Jenny is 'Ken' (not the stereotypical fashion dolls, you understand! Her Ken is a Neanderthal cockney 'bloke' and I play 'Barbie' as a posh Conservative 'lady' trying to educate the ignorant fool!) and we mess around and have fun with our voices. [Laughs]

J: We didn't do that before. I love it. Life's not easy but we are there for each other. We sing, laugh and cry together. We really do...

Soft tears. Embracing. Laughter ripples, and floats up into London's night sky...

Applied Improvisation Games

Below are descriptions of the small selection of games we have included in this book. They are listed in the order they appear in Chapter 4.

For more improv games see: *The Improv Encyclopaedia*[1] and Robbins Dudeck, T. and McClure, C. (eds) (2018) *Applied Improvisation: Leading, Collaborating and Creating beyond the Theatre*. London: Bloomsbury Methuen Drama.

FACILITATION

A general proviso for the inclusion of games and other whole body work is to ensure that facilitators adapt them in advance for the diversity of physical and other needs, and that participants are clear that they are free to join in as they choose. Use demonstration where necessary to help set the rules of the game.

Some suggestions are given for facilitating the debrief, but it is recommended that very little is said to put any 'spin' on the purpose of a game before experiencing it. This allows more of the participants' own experiencing and reflection to emerge in the debrief. Debrief can elicit what participants are taking from learning about self, and from observing others, into everyday vocal situations.

PRE-NAME-LINE-UP
(from random sitting/standing)

It can be less pressure to break the ice *before* the learning of names and sharing of personal information, and we like to minimize the use

---

1   http://improvencyclopedia.org

of name labels. Line-ups are also useful for getting everyone moving, releasing physical tension, and talking freely early on. This game is played from a random sitting/standing position.

We avoid anything that might focus on physical appearance for obvious reasons. Participants are given about 30 seconds (be creative with time monitoring here!) to line up according to, for example:

- what time you went to bed last night, earliest to latest

- the month and date of your birthday, with 1 January one end, and 31 December the other

- shortest and longest journey either in terms of distance or travel time

- the last time you made a phone call.

At the end of the time limit, dates and times are called out in sequence to see if it follows a chronological order.

BALL NAME GAMES
(in a circle)

Round 1: Participants say their own name then throw a ball across the circle to the next participant who catches it then repeats. On balance, people like a prop, and at an early stage this encourages eye contact with another group member, and can release tension through making it okay to laugh when the ball is dropped.

Round 2 option: Participants say their own name then throw to someone else whose name they remember. They can simply ask if they have forgotten.

Round 3 option: The group repeats Round 1 aiming to throw to and name the next peer in the same order.

NAME AND BREAKFAST
(in a circle)

This operates as Rounds 1 and 3 above, with participants adding their favourite breakfast food after their name. Remembering name plus breakfast food is harder but sharing some simple personal information in this way can be freeing and helps in focusing attention out on others.

ALLITERATION NAME
(in a circle)

The first volunteer says their own name to the person on their right; this second person says their own name plus introduces the first person to the person on *their* right, adding a positive alliterative attribute, and so on, for example 'I'm Jo, and this is Amiable Ali', 'I'm Sam and this is Jaunty Jo'. Facilitators and other group members can prompt attributes where necessary.

UPSIDE-DOWN INTRODUCTIONS
(in pairs then feedback to the circle)

For a more straightforward and sedate 'getting to know you' exercise that breaks up the circle, members can simply have time in pairs to share names, a passion and some other piece of information – where they have travelled from, if not used in the initial warm-up. The 'upside-down' element is simply one person having to introduce and share information on their partner back to the whole group and vice versa.

1,2,3
(in pairs)

Initial demonstration is definitely helpful here.

Round 1: In pairs, the objective is to count to 3 repeatedly, alternating numbers from one partner to the other, so:

A 1
B 2
A 3
B 1
A 2
B 3 and so on.

Start again if a mistake is made. Allow the game to continue for long enough for some pairs to make mistakes, laugh, etc.

Short debrief on how easy it was (often harder than people expected) and what helped success (especially focusing attention) before moving on to Round 2. Introduce the idea that we are disrupting a familiar mental map to introduce a new skill pattern and that practice helps establish this.

Round 2: Same pairs repeat the exercise, replacing the number 2 with a clap, so:

A 1
B clap
A 3
B 1
A clap
B 3 and so on.

Again, a short debrief to elicit whether this was easier or harder, and what helped. Comment on observations that people slowed down, used more eye contact, laughed if a mistake was made, if these are not shared spontaneously. People will often say that getting into a rhythm helped, and possibly that this round is easier as the clap breaks up automatic number sequencing.

Round 3: An option to include a third round in which the number 3 is replaced by a movement or gesture. This is fun, but doesn't add much in our view in the debrief, apart from encouraging spontaneous movement, giving the opportunity to debrief self-consciousness and using voice as part of the whole body in communication.

WHAT ARE YOU DOING?
(in a circle)

This game also introduces body movement and nonverbal communication in addition to emphasizing pitch patterns for intonation in questions and responses.

It can either be played in a circle, passing round the question/response one way in turn, or with increased challenge by a participant stepping into the centre of the circle and then anyone can volunteer to step in, respond with the question, and take over to do a new mime.

A begins a simple everyday mime.

B asks (use name) 'A, what are you doing?'

A responds *verbally* with a completely different everyday activity from the one still being mimed.

B mimes the new action that is verbally described.

C asks 'B, what are you doing?'

B responds *verbally* with a completely different everyday activity from the mimed one.

And so on....

For example:

A mimes washing face.

B: 'A, what are you doing?'

A continues to mime washing face and says 'I'm packing a suitcase.'

B: 'Oh' and mimes packing a suitcase.

C: 'B, what are you doing?'

B continues to mime packing a suitcase and says 'I'm stroking the cat.'

And so on......

The additional rule is that participants practise using different intonation patterns for the question 'What are you doing?' to infer different meanings.

YES NO
(in a circle)

A says 'Yes' to participant B on their left.

B chooses either to pass 'Yes' on to the next person on their left, C, or to return a 'No' to A on their right.

Recipient A or C chooses a Yes or No response,

'Yes' always travels to the left and 'No' to the right.

Additional rule: each person must vary the vocal dynamics from the one before, in terms of pitch movement, loudness, voice quality, pace, thus intonation and inferred meaning change.

NAME AND YOUR SUPERPOWER
(in pairs or a circle)

It is useful to re-visit a name game in Session 2 as there has usually been a three- or four-week gap. Staying in a circle can require more courage and spontaneity, and focuses attention on the wider group.

Superpowers can be as general as you wish, or focused on the present moment.

PRESIDENT-BODYGUARD
(usually standing in pairs, but fine
if participants need to sit)

This can be simplified to a physical mirroring game, or to just mirroring speech.

Pairs decide who is A and who is B. A is the president and B the bodyguard who must protect the president from any assassins.

The bodyguard does this by mirroring the president as closely to real-time as possible, so that an assassin would not be able to tell who is the president and who the bodyguard at any given moment.

The president starts to speak and use gesture slowly and the bodyguard begins to copy.

Facilitators should demonstrate and then support the presidents in using strategies such as drawn-out vowels, and exaggerated intonation, to be as helpful as possible (they don't want to get assassinated!). Participants may otherwise try to catch their partner out by going too quickly, or not know how to draw out speech.

Allow this to continue for 2 or 3 minutes, then the pairs swap roles (you could also swap pairs around to mix the group up).

Debrief often elicits the intense focus on the other person, using eye contact, and on their own lips, sounds and voice. Facilitators can link to empathy and the collaborative effort to succeed, and to aspects of emotional intelligence that will be explored during later voice and communication exercises.

(TELEPHONE) CHINESE WHISPERS
(designed for a larger group but can
be adapted for small numbers)

This explores gist recall and perception, interpreting the meaning and emotion of others' communication.

We sometimes use this as a rehearsal for 'Hot telephone', so it is described in this way below, but it could be simply passing on a story.

The group is in a circle with two chairs as the 'hot seats' for A and B, and a barrier/screen between them.

C goes out of the room.

A tells B a short personal story that has some emotional content (facilitate people to only disclose what they are happy to, possibly offering excitement, anger or surprise as their emotional content). The conversation is role-played as if over the phone.

C is called back into the room.

B relates the gist of the 'phone call' to C, aiming to convey the emotional tone and vocal expression they heard.

PRESENT IN MY POCKET
(two lines, facing each other and opposite a partner)

This is a good game for managing self-consciousness in playing with pitch and intonation, smile tone, and so on.

It is another good rehearsal for using more overt signals on the telephone.

Round 1: As walk at the same time towards their partner Bs, pulling an imaginary present out of a pocket, saying: 'I've got you a present' using pitch initiation, smile tone and additional bounce for excitement

B responds with 'Oh' using thin fold surprise.

A says 'It's a ....', choosing what the present is

B responds with 'Thank you/thanks very much' possibly adding a short statement such as 'How lovely' 'What a surprise' 'That's really great/kind of you'.

The responses can fit an appropriate level of practice, from single words, to formulaic statements of gratitude and surprise.

Repeat, with A and B swapping roles.

Round 2 option: the present is something that would not normally be pleasant.

B has to respond with an authentic polite rejection.

Some examples of presents might include: a bucket of slimy snails; a dirty hankie; a rotting fish; some dead flowers.

Some examples of response might include:

- 'Oh, that's not what I expected.'

- 'It's kind of you to think of me, but you keep it.'

- 'Thanks, but unfortunately I can't accept it.'

- 'Thank you, but unfortunately I don't eat...'

Again, A and B swap roles.

Debrief what people heard and saw in terms of vocal and

communication dynamics. What might they usefully play with and use on the telephone?

POSITIVE-NEGATIVE
(in pairs)
Participants are in A/B pairs.

A starts a conversation with a positive emotional tone and language.

B responds, keeping on the same topic, but with a 'negative' emotional tone and language.

A responds, switching the tone back to positive.

After a few minutes, A/B switch roles and A begins a new topic, thus both experience a different emotion.

Debrief can highlight the difference and what was used to maintain positive emotion. In addition, discussion about the challenge of keeping our voice tone positive when the other is perceived as negative may be useful. This can link to the challenge of maintaining new vocal skills, such as using more pitch changes in intonation, when the listener has a flatter pattern and is using lower pitch.

STORY ONE-WORD-AT-A-TIME
(in a circle)
One person starts the story with only the first word.

The story continues to build around the circle only one word at a time until the group decides it concludes.

The sentences have to make sense grammatically but can be as wild as the group wishes in terms of content.

Participants are encouraged to use the previous word to build rather than try and predict where the sentence or whole story is going.

Participants are encouraged to use intonation to bring meaning and expression, and use pause although not overthink their choice of word to add to the story.

Debrief can be around managing being spontaneous and freer, allowing any response, and collaborative dialogue. It is also useful to highlight the challenge of maintaining a personal voice goal in addition to the cognitive demand of the game.

TAKES ME TO THE TIME WHEN...
(in a circle)

The facilitator gives a word to the first person, for example 'suitcase' (the word does not have to be a noun).

That person responds with: 'Suitcase takes me to to the time when...' and completes with any personal memory of 'suitcase', for example: 'Suitcase takes me to the time when I left my suitcase on a train'. The statement must be true for the speaker, even if it results in them saying 'I have never seen an X'.

The speaker then gives a new word to the person on their left to respond to.

Step up the challenge by throwing a ball to someone across the circle, so the order is not predictable.

Participants can aim to be using a personal voice goal in just the first formulaic phrase, or being more consistent across the story.

Debrief around managing anxiety of waiting your turn, and self-consciousness and pressure to respond, in addition to the challenge of honest, personal disclosure.

WAITING ROOM
(in a circle)

We use this game as a role-play for experiencing being present and managing anxiety.

We are in a doctor's waiting room.

One volunteer, A, leaves the room and the group decides where the empty chair should be.

One person, B, sitting adjacent to the empty chair, is chosen to respond.

A re-enters the room and has to:

- pause and 'take their space'

- look around the circle for the empty chair

- choose a way of asking whether the seat is free, whether anyone is sitting there, whether it is okay to sit down, etc.

B chooses to respond with either yes or no.

A responds in turn and may choose to negotiate.

The game repeats with a different volunteer leaving the room.

Step up: B chooses their response and the person the other side of the empty chair, C, presents a challenge to this, for example:

A: Excuse me, is this chair free?

B: Yes, sure no problem.

C: Actually, I'm keeping this for my Dad who's a bit late.

A: I'm being called in in just a few minutes, so are you okay if I just sit there until then?

A has to respond, managing both speakers.

Debrief includes how it felt to enter the room, take space, pause and engage with others to make a request assertively rather than apologetically.

In addition, strategies for managing rejection, conflict and persuasion are explored.

THE ORACLE
(whole group sitting)

This is similar to 'Story one-word-at-a-time', with more focus on collaborative listening and a particular topic. It is also great fun. It works best with a group large enough to have several volunteers and several in the audience, so around six minimum, or adapt as appropriate.

At least three volunteers become 'The oracle' – wise and all-knowing.

Someone in the audience calls out a word to define that is related to voice and communication and to strategies practised in the group, for example resonance, hum-pitch.

'The oracle' gives a definition, with each person taking turns to add one word until a collaborative conclusion is reached.

Again, the practice is to stay open and listen to what has gone before, letting go of one's own preconceived sentence and making something new together.

'The oracle' can be adapted for a smaller group by having a selection of words on cards to pick from rather than an audience. Having the opportunity to listen to and observe the oracle, however, is fun and provides rich material for debrief discussion in terms of dialogue and transferable skills.

References

Adler, R.K., Hirsch, S. and Pickering, J. (eds) (2018) *Voice and Communication Therapy for the Transgender/Gender Diverse Client: A Comprehensive Clinical Guide* (3rd edn). San Diego, CA: Plural Publishing.

Azul, D. (2015) 'Transmasculine people's vocal situations: a critical review of gender-related discourses and empirical data.' *International Journal of Language & Communication Disorders, 50*(1), 31–47. https://doi.org/10.1111/1460-6984.12121

Azul, D., Nygren, U., Södersten, M. and Neuschaefer-Rube, C. (2017) 'Transmasculine people's voice function: a review of the currently available evidence.' *Journal of Voice, 31*(2), 261.e9–261.e23. https://doi.org/10.1016/j.jvoice.2016.05.005

Baker, J. (2017) *Psychosocial Perspectives on the Management of Voice Disorders: Implications for Patients and Clients, Options and Strategies for Clinicians.* Oxford: Compton Publishing.

Barker, M. (2013) *Mindful Counselling and Psychotherapy: Practising Mindfully Across Approaches and Issues.* London: Sage Publications Ltd.

Barker, M.-J. (2018) 'Trans: Adventurers Across Time and Space' blog. 13 November. Accessed on 22/11/2019 at www.rewriting-the-rules.com/gender/trans-time-and-space/

Barker, M.-J. and Iantaffi, A. (2019) *Life Isn't Binary: On Being Both, Beyond, and In-Between.* London: Jessica Kingsley Publishers.

Barker, M.-J. and Scheele, J. (2016) *Queer: A Graphic History.* London: Icon Books Ltd.

Barrett, J. (2017) 'Gender dysphoria: assessment and management for non-specialists.' *BMJ.* https://doi.org/10.1136/bmj.j2866

Beattie, M. and Lenihan, P. with Dundas, R. (2018) *Counselling Skills for Working with Gender Diversity and Identity.* London: Jessica Kingsley Publishers.

Berne, E. (2010) *Games People Play.* London: Penguin.

Berry, C. (1994) *Your Voice and How to Use It* (revised edn). London: Virgin Books.

Betancourt, J.R. (2003) 'Defining cultural competence: a practical framework for addressing racial/ethnic disparities in health and health care.' *Public Health Reports, 118*(4), 293–302. https://doi.org/10.1093/phr/118.4.293

Block, C., Papp, V.G. and Adler, R.K. (2019) 'Transmasculine Voice and Communication.' In R.K. Adler, S. Hirsch and J. Pickering (eds) *Voice and Communication Therapy for the Transgender/Gender Diverse Client: A Comprehensive Clinical Guide.* San Diego, CA: Plural Publishing.

Bogost, I. (2016) *Play Anything: The Pleasure of Limits, the Use of Boredom, and the Secret of Games.* New York: Basic Books.

Bonenfant, Y. (2010) 'Queer listening to queer vocal timbres.' *Performance Research, 15*(3), 74–80.

Boston, J. (2018) *Voice: Readings in Theatre Practice.* London: Palgrave.

Brown, B. (2018) *Daring Greatly: How the Courage to Be Vulnerable Transforms the Way We Live, Love, Parent, and Lead.* London: Penguin Books Ltd.

Burns, C. (2019) *Trans Britain: Our Journey from the Shadows.* London: Unbound.

Butcher, P., Elias, A. and Cavalli, L. (2007) *Understanding and Treating Psychogenic Voice Disorder: A CBT Framework.* Chichester: John Wiley & Sons.

Campbell, P., Constantino, C. and Simpson, S. (eds) (2019) *Stammering Pride and Prejudice: Difference Not Defect.* Guilford: J & R Press.

Caughter, S. and Crofts, V. (2018) 'Nurturing a resilient mindset in school-aged children who stutter.' *American Journal of Speech-Language Pathology, 27,* 1111–1123.

Carey, D. and Carey R. (2008) *The Vocal Arts Workbook: A Practical Course for Developing the Expressive Range of Your Voice.* London: Bloomsbury Methuen Drama.

Cheasman, C., Everard, R. and Simpson, S. (2013) *Stammering Therapy from the Inside : New Perspectives on Working with Young People and Adults.* Guilford: J & R Press Ltd.

Coutu, D. (2002) How Resilience Works. *Harvard Business Review,* May. Accessed on 26/11/2019 at https://hbr.org/2002/05/how-resilience-works

Crenshaw, K. (1989) 'Demarginalizing the intersection of race and sex: a Black feminist critique of antidiscrimination doctrine, feminist theory and antiracist politics.' *University of Chicago Legal Forum, 1*(8), 139–167. Accessed on 26/11/2019 at https://chicagounbound.uchicago.edu/cgi/viewcontent.cgi?article=1052&context=uclf

Davidson, S., Mills, M., Bracken, C., Stoneham and Moos, M. (2019) 'Voice and communication at family day: a collaboration between GIDS and London

GIC.' Presented at the British Association of Gender Identity Specialists 5th Symposium, Durham, 3–4 October 2019.

Davies, S., Papp, V. and Antoni, C. (2015) 'Voice and communication for gender nonconforming individuals: giving voice to the person inside.' *International Journal of Transgenderism, 16*(3), 117–159.

de Shazer, S., Dolan, M., Korman, H., Trepper, T., McCollum, E. and Berg, I.K. (2012) *More Than Miracles: The State of the Art of Solution-Focused Brief Therapy* (2nd edn). New York: Routledge.

Denborough, D. (2014) *Retelling the Stories of Our Lives: Everyday Narrative Therapy to Draw Inspiration and Transform Experience.* New York: W.W. Norton.

D'haeseleer, E., Bettens, K., Corthals, P. and Cosyns, M. (2019) 'Acoustic and perceptual effects of articulation exercises in trans women.' Presented at the European Professional Association of Transgender Health (EPATH), Rome, 11–13 April 2019.

DiLollo, A. and Favreau, C. (2010) 'Person-centered care and speech and language therapy.' *Seminars in Speech and Language, 31*(02), 090–097. https://doi.org/10.1055/s-0030-1252110

DiLollo, A. and Neimeyer, R.A. (2014) *Counseling in Speech-Language Pathology and Audiology: Reconstructing Personal Narratives.* San Diego, CA: Plural Publishing Inc.

do Mar Pereira, M. (2017) *Power, Knowledge and Feminist Scholarship: An Ethnography of Academia.* London: Routledge.

Duffy, P. (ed.) 2015 *A Reflective Practitioner's Guide to (mis)Adventures in Drama Education – or – What Was I Thinking?* Bristol: Intellect.

Dundas, R. (2018) 'Shame, Stigma and Trans People.' In M. Beattie and P. Lenihan with R. Dundas, *Counselling Skills for Working with Gender Diversity and Identity.* London: Jessica Kingsley Publishers.

Epston, D. and White, M. (1992) 'Consulting Your Consultants: The Documentations of Alternative Knowledges.' In D. Epston and M. White, *Experience Contradiction, Narrative and Imagination: Selected Papers of David Epston and Michael White, 1989–1991.* Adelaide: Dulwich Centre Publications.

Feldman, C. and Kuyken, W. (2019) *Mindfulness: Ancient Wisdom Meets Modern Psychology.* New York: The Guilford Press.

Fife, S.T., Whiting, J.B., Bradford, K. and Davis, S. (2013) 'The therapeutic pyramid: a common factors synthesis of techniques, alliance, and way of being.' *Journal of Marital and Family Therapy, 40*(1), 20–33. https://doi.org/10.1111/jmft.12041

Flasher, L.V. and Fogle, P.T. (2012) *Counseling Skills for Speech-Language Pathologists and Audiologists* (2nd edn). Clifton Park: Delmar.

Fourie, R. (2009) 'Qualitative study of the therapeutic relationship in speech and language therapy: perspectives of adults with acquired communication and swallowing disorders.' *International Journal of Language & Communication Disorders, 44*(6), 979–999. https://doi.org/10.3109/13682820802535285

Fox, H. (2003) 'Using therapeutic documents: a review.' *The International Journal of Narrative Therapy and Community Work, 4*, 26–36.

Frost, A. and Yarrow, R. (2016) *Improvisation in Drama, Theatre and Performance : History, Practice, Theory.* London: Palgrave.

Gilbert, P. (2015) *The Compassionate Mind: A New Approach to Life's Challenges.* London: Robinson.

Glickstein, L. (1998) *Be Heard Now! Tap into Your Inner Speaker and Communicate with Ease.* New York: Broadway Books.

Goleman, D. (2009) *Working with Emotional Intelligence.* New York: Bantam Books.

Goyder, C. (2014) *Gravitas: Communicate with Confidence, Influence and Authority.* London: Vermilion.

Hancock, A.B., Childs, K.D. and Irwig, M.S. (2017) 'Trans male voice in the first year of testosterone therapy: make no assumptions.' *Journal of Speech, Language and Hearing Research, 60*, 2472–2482. https://doi.org/10.1044/2017_JSLHR-S-16-0320

Hancock, A.B. and Siegfriedt, L. (2020) *Transforming Voice and Communication with Transgender and Gender-Diverse People: An Evidence-Based Process.* San Diego, CA: Plural Publishing.

Harley, J. (2015) 'Bridging the gap between cognitive therapy and acceptance and commitment therapy (ACT).' *Procedia – Social and Behavioral Sciences,193*, 131–140.

Harley, J. (2018) 'The role of attention in therapy for children and adolescents who stutter: cognitive behavioral therapy and mindfulness-based interventions.' *American Journal of Speech-Language Pathology, 27*, 1139–1151.

Harris, R. (2007) *The Happiness Trap.* London: Robinson.

Higgs, J., Jones, M., Loftus, S. and Christensen, N. (2008) *Clinical Reasoning in the Health Professions* (3rd edn). Philadelphia, PA: Elsevier.

Hoby, H. (2011) 'Justin Bond: "I think everybody's trans."' *The Guardian*, 28 June, 2011. Accessed on 13/11/2019 at www.theguardian.com/stage/2011/jun/28/justin-bond

Hogan, C. (2018) *The Alchemy of Performance Anxiety: Transformation for Artists.* London: Free Association Books.

Houseman, B. (2002) *Finding Your Voice: A Complete Voice Training Manual for Actors.* London: Nick Hern Books.

Hughes, R. (2016) *Time-Limited Art Psychotherapy: Developments in Theory and Practice.* London: Routledge.

Iantaffi, A. and Barker, M-J. (2018) *How to Understand Your Gender: A Practical Guide for Exploring Who You Are*. London: Jessica Kingsley Publishers

Irons, C. (2019) *Compassionate Mind Approach to Emotional Difficulties: Using Compassion-Focused Therapy*. London: Robinson.

Irons, C. and Beaumont, E. (2017) *Compassionate Mind Workbook*. London: Robinson.

Iveson, C., George, E. and Ratner, H. (2012) *Brief Coaching: A Solution Focused Approach*. New York: Routledge.

Jackson, P.Z. (2015) *Easy: Your LIFEPASS to Creativity and Confidence*. London: The Solutions Focus.

James, S. and Brumfitt, S. (2018) *Applying Psychological Ideas in Speech and Language Therapy*. Guildford: J & R Press.

Kabat-Zinn, J. (1990) *Full Catastrophe Living*. London: Piatkus.

Kabat-Zinn, J. (2016) *Mindfulness for Beginners: Reclaiming the Present Moment and Your Life*. Boulder, CO: Sounds True.

Karpman, S.B. (1968) 'Fairy tales and script drama analysis.' *Transactional Analysis Bulletin, 26*(7), 39–43.

Karpman, S.B. (2014) *A Game Free Life: The Definitive Book on the Drama Triangle and the Compassion Triangle by the Originator and Author*. San Francisco, CA: Drama Triangle Productions.

Kay, K. and Shipman, C. (2014) *The Confidence Code: The Science and Art of Self-Assurance – What Women Should Know*. New York: Harper Collins Publishers.

Kelman, E. and Wheeler, S. (2015) 'Cognitive behavioral therapy with children who stutter.' *Procedia – Social and Behavioral Sciences,193*, 165–174.

Kermis, M.H. and Goldman, B.M. (2006) 'A multicomponent conceptualization of authenticity: theory and research.' *Advances in Experimental Social Psychology, 38*, 285–357.

Kirmayer, L.J. (2012) 'Rethinking cultural competence.' *Transcultural Psychiatry, 49*(2), 149–164. https://doi.org/10.1177/1363461512444673

Kitson, A., Harvey, G. and McCormack, B. (1998) 'Enabling the implementation of evidence based practice: a conceptual framework.' *Quality and Safety in Health Care, 7*(3), 149–158. https://doi.org/10.1136/qshc.7.3.149

Leahy, M.M., O'Dwyer, M. and Ryan, F. (2012) 'Witnessing stories: Definitional Ceremonies in Narrative Therapy with adults who stutter.' *Journal of Fluency Disorders, 37*(4), 234–241. https://doi.org/10.1016/j.jfludis.2012.03.001

Lester, C. (2018) CN Lester on inclusive feminism: all about women 2018. YouTube Video. Accessed on 21/11/2019 at www.youtube.com/watch?v=5a5S6fv-m80

Lester, C.N. (2017) *Trans Like Me: A Journey for All of Us*. London: Virago.

Linklater, C. (2006) *Freeing the Natural Voice* (2nd revised edn). London: Nick Hern Books.

Logan, J. (2013) 'New Stories of Stammering: A Narrative Approach.' In C. Cheasman, R. Everard and S. Simpson (eds) *Stammering Therapy from the Inside*. Guildford: J& R Press.

Lorde, A. (1984/2019) *Sister Outsider*. London: Penguin Classics.

Lucy, D., Poorkavoos, M. and Thompson, A. (2014) *Building Resilience: Five Key Capabilities*. London: Roffey Park Institute Ltd.

Malchiodi, C.A. (2012) *Handbook of Art Therapy* (2nd edn). New York: Guilford Press.

Malchiodi, C.A. (2018) *Handbook of Art Therapy and Digital Technology*. London: Jessica Kingsley Publishers.

McGilchrist, I. (2009/2019) *The Master and His Emissary: The Divided Brain and the Making of the Western World*. New Haven, CT: Yale University Press.

McLaren, P. (2016) *Life in Schools: An Introduction to Critical Pedagogy in the Foundations of Education*. London: Routledge.

Martin, S and Darnley, L. (2017) *The Voice in Education*. Braunton, Devon: Compton Publishing Ltd.

Martinez, L.R., Sawyer, K.B., Thoroughgood, C.N., Ruggs, E.N. and Smith, N.A. (2017) 'The importance of being "me": the relation between authentic identity expression and transgender employees' work related attitudes and experiences.' *Journal of Applied Psychology, 102*(2), 215–226.

Mearns, D., Thorne, B. with Mcleod, J. (2013) *Person-Centred Counselling in Action* (4th edn). London: Sage.

Meyer, I. H. (2003) 'Prejudice, social stress, and mental health in lesbian, gay, and bisexual populations: conceptual issues and research evidence.' *Psychological Bulletin, 129*(5), 674–697. https://doi.org/10.1037/0033-2909.129.5.674

Mguni, N., Bacon, N. and Brown, J. (2014) *The Wellbeing and Resilience Paradox*. London: The Young Foundation.

Michie, S., Atkins, L and West, R. (2014) *The Behaviour Change Wheel: A Guide to Designing Interventions*. Sutton: Silverback Publishing.

Mills, M. (2015) 'Lived experience of voice: a service evaluation of the voice group programme at Charing Cross Gender Identity Clinic.' Presented at the European Professional Association of Transgender Health (EPATH), Ghent, 12–14 March 2015.

Mills, M. (2016) 'The client as expert: using Narrative Therapy ideas and practices to support voice and communication group therapy for trans women to 're-author' their stories of communicative competence and preferred vocal identity.' Presented at the World Professional Association of Transgender Health (WPATH), Amsterdam, 17–21 June 2016.

Mills, M. and Gorb, N. (2017) 'Charting the unknown: new client outcomes and journeys of vocal identity.' Presented at the British Association of Gender Identity Specialists 3rd Symposium, Glasgow, 5–6 October 2016.

Mills, M., Stoneham, G., Bracken, C., Gorb, N. and Davies, S. (2019a) 'At the cutting edge: towards a new terminology and understanding of voice and communication for non-binary people.' Presented at the European Professional Association of Transgender Health (EPATH), Rome, 11–13 April 2019.

Mills, M., Stoneham, G. and Davies, S. (2019b) 'Toward a protocol for transmasculine voice: a service evaluation of the voice and communication therapy group program, including long-term follow-up for trans men at the London Gender Identity Clinic.' *Transgender Health 4*, 1. https://doi.org/10.1089/trgh.2019.0011

Mills, M. and Stoneham, G. (2016) 'Giving voice to our transgender clients: developing competency and co-working.' *Royal College of Speech and Language Therapists Bulletin* (July).

Mills, M., and Stoneham, G. (2017) *The Voice Book for Trans and Non-Binary People: A Practical Guide to Creating and Sustaining Authentic Voice and Communication*. London: Jessica Kingsley Publishers.

Mills, M., Stoneham, G. and Georgiadou, I. (2017) 'Expanding the evidence: developments and innovations in clinical practice, training and competency within voice and communication therapy for trans and gender diverse people.' *International Journal of Transgenderism, 18*(3), 328–342. https://doi.org/10.1080/15532739.2017.1329049

Mills, M., Stoneham, G., Kurji-Smith, N., Gorb, N. and Elias, A. (2018) 'New horizons: responding to service demand.' *Royal College of Speech and Language Therapists Bulletin* (February).

Moon, B.L. (2016) *Art-Based Group Therapy: Theory and Practice* (2nd edn). Springfield, IL: Charles C. Thomas.

Nelson, J. (2017) *The Voice Exercise Book*. London: Nick Hern Books.

Nirta, C. (2018) *Marginal Bodies, Trans Utopias*. London: Routledge.

Nygren, U., Nordenskjöld, A., Arver, S. and Södersten, M. (2016) 'Effects on voice fundamental frequency and satisfaction with voice in trans men during testosterone treatment: a longitudinal study.' *Journal of Voice, 30*, 766.e23–766.e34.

Oates, J.M. (2019) 'Evidence-Based Practice in Voice Training for Trans Women.' In R.K. Adler, S. Hirsch and J. Pickering (eds) *Voice and Communication Therapy for the Transgender/Gender Diverse Client: A Comprehensive Clinical Guide*. San Diego, CA: Plural Publishing.

Ochsner, K. and Gross, J. (2004) 'Thinking Makes It So: Social Cognitive Neuroscience Approach to Emotional Regulation.' In R. Baumeister and

K. Vohs (eds) *The Handbook of Self-Regulation: Research, Theory and Applications*. London: The Guilford Press.

Patel, N. (2017) 'Violent cistems: trans experiences of bathroom space.' *Agenda*, *31*(1), 51–63. https://doi.org/10.1080/10130950.2017.1369717

Paul, A.M. (2012) 'What the jazz greats knew about creativity.' *Psychology Today*. Accessed on 21/11/2019 at www.psychologytoday.com/blog/how-be-brilliant/201206/what-the-jazz-greats-knew-about-creativity

Pearce, R. (2018) *Understanding Trans Health*. Bristol: Policy Press.

Pert, S. (2019) 'Talking loud and clear.' *Bulletin: Magazine of the Royal College of Speech and Language Therapists*, June, 16–18.

Poynton, R. (2013) *Do Improvise: Less Push. More Pause. Better Results. A New Approach to Work (and Life)*. London: The Do Book Company.

Prendiville, P. (2008) *Developing Facilitation Skills: A Handbook for Group Facilitators* (2nd edn). Dublin: Combat Poverty Agency.

Preston, A.M., and TEDx Talks (2018) 'Effective Allyship: A Transgender Take on Intersectionality.' Youtube video. Accessed on 13/11/2019 at www.youtube.com/watch?v=3EcuDfDjUd8

Preston, S. (2016) *Applied Theatre: Facilitation: Pedagogies, Practices, Resilience*. London: Bloomsbury Methuen Drama.

RCSLT (Royal College of Speech and Language Therapists) (2018) *Trans and Gender Diverse Voice and Communication Therapy Competency Framework*. London: RCSLT.

Redstone, A. (2004) 'Researching people's experience of narrative therapy: acknowledging the contribution of the "client" to what works in counselling conversations.' *International Journal of Narrative Therapy and Community Work*, *2*, 1–6.

Richards, C., Arcelus, J., Barrett, J., Bouman, W. P. *et al.* (2015) 'Trans is not a disorder – but should still receive funding.' *Sexual and Relationship Therapy*, *30*(3), 309–313. https://doi.org/10.1080/14681994.2015.1054110

Richards, C. and Barker, M. (2013) *Sexuality and Gender for Mental Health Professionals: A Practical Guide*. London: Sage.

Richards, C., Barker, M., Lenihan, P. and Iantaffi, A. (2014) 'Who watches the watchmen? A critical perspective on the theorization of trans people and clinicians.' *Feminism and Psychology*, *24*(2), 248–258. https://doi.org/10.1177/0959353514526220

Richards, C., Bouman, W.P. and Barker, M.-J. (2017) *Genderqueer and Non-Binary Genders*. London: Palgrave Macmillan.

Robbins Dudeck, T. and McClure, C. (2018) *Applied Improvisation: Leading, Collaborating and Creating beyond the Theatre*. London: Bloomsbury Methuen Drama.

Roche, J. (2018) *Queer Sex: A Trans and Non-Binary Guide to Intimacy, Pleasure and Relationships*. London: Jessica Kingsley Publishers.

Roche, J. (2020) *Trans Power: Own Your Gender*. London: Jessica Kingsley Publishers.

Rodenburg, P. (2009) *Power Presentation: Formal Speech in an Informal World*. London: Michael Joseph Books.

Rodenburg, P. (2015) *The Right To Speak*. (2nd revised edn). London: Bloomsbury Methuen Drama.

Rodenburg, P. (2017) *The Second Circle: Using Positive Energy for Success in Every Situation* (reprinted edn). New York: W.W. Norton & Company.

Rogers, C.R. (2004) *On Becoming a Person: A Therapist's View of Psychotherapy*. London: Constable & Robinson.

Rogers, J. (2010) *Facilitating Groups*. Maidenhead: McGraw-Hill/Open University Press.

Schön, D.A. (1987/2014) *Educating the Reflective Practitioner: Toward a New Design for Teaching and Learning in the Professions*. San Francisco, CA: Jossey-Bass.

Seal, L. and Higgison, C. (2019) 'Becoming competent: new professional training pathways in gender dysphoria care in the UK.' Presented at the British Association of Gender Identity Specialists 5th Symposium, Durham, 3–4 October 2019.

Segal, Z.V., Williams, M. and Teasdale, J.D. (2018) *Mindfulness-Based Cognitive Therapy for Depression* (2nd edn). New York: The Guilford Press.

Seligman, M.E.P. (2011) Building Resilience. Harvard Business Review, April. Accessed on 18/11/2019 at https://hbr.org/2011/04/building-resilience

Sharpe, A. (2019) 'Sexual Intimacy, Gender Identity and "Fraud".' Presented at the European Professional Association of Transgender Health, Rome, 11–13 April 2019.

Shennan, G. (2014) *Solution-Focused Practice: Effective Communication to Facilitate Change*. London: Palgrave.

Shennan, G. and Iveson, C. (2008) 'What difference would that make?' *Journal of Family Psychotherapy*, *19*(1), 97–101. https://doi.org/10.1080/08975350801904254

Shennan, G. and Iveson, C. (2011) 'From Solution to Description: Practice and Research in Tandem.' In C. Franklin, T.S. Trepper, E.E. McCollum and W.J. Gingerich (eds) *Solution-Focused Brief Therapy: A Handbook of Evidence-Based Practice*. New York: Oxford University Press.

Shewell, C. (2009) *Voice Work: Art and Science in Changing Voices*. Chichester: Wiley-Blackwell.

Shewell, C. (2013) 'Listening properly.' *Royal College of Speech and Language Therapists Bulletin* (July).

Slaski, M. and Cartwright, S. (2003) 'Emotional intelligence training and its implications for stress, health and performance.' *Stress and Health, 19*(4), 233–239. https://doi.org/10.1002/smi.979

Smythe, V. (2018) 'I'm credited with having coined the word "Terf". Here's how it happened.' Accessed on 21 January 2020 at www.theguardian.com/commentisfree/2018/nov/29/im-credited-with-having-coined-the-acronym-terf-heres-how-it-happened

Sontag, S. (2009) *Styles of Radical Will.* London: Penguin Books.

Steinhauer, K., Klimek, M.M. and Estill, J. (2017) *The Estill Voice Model: Theory and Translation.* Pittsburgh, KS: Estill Voice International.

Stemple, J.C. and Hapner, E.R. (2014) *Voice Therapy: Clinical Case Studies* (4th edn). San Diego, CA: Plural Publishing.

Stoneham, G. (2015) 'Sing for Your Life: Establishing a transgender voice group: benefits for students and clients.' Presented at the European Professional Association of Transgender Health, Ghent, 12–14 March 2015.

Teasdale, J.D. and Chaskalson (Kulananda), M. (2011) 'How does mindfulness transform suffering? II: the transformation ofdukkha.' *Contemporary Buddhism, 12*(1), 103–124. https://doi.org/10.1080/14639947.2011.564826

Tellis, C.M. and Barone, O.R. (2016) *Counseling and Interviewing in Speech-Language Pathology and Audiology: A Therapy Resource.* Burlington, MA: Jones & Bartlett Learning.

Tellyjuice (2018) *The Second Train.* Accessed on 22/11/2019 at https://vimeo.com/289072627

Tervalon, M. and Murray-Garcia, J. (1998) 'Cultural humility versus cultural competence: a critical distinction in defining physician training outcomes in multicultural education.' *Journal of Health Care for the Poor and Underserved, 9*(2), 117–125.

Thomas, G. (2008) 'Facilitate first thyself: the person-centered dimension of facilitator education.' *Journal of Experiential Education, 31*(2), 168–188. https://doi.org/10.5193/jee.31.2.168

Titze, I.R. (2006) 'Voice Training and Therapy with semi-occluded vocal tract: rationale and scientific underpinnings.'*Journal of Speech Language & Hearing Research, 49*(2),448–459.

Titze, I.R. and Verdolini Abbott, K. (2012) *Vocology: The Science and Practice of Voice Habilitation.* Salt Lake City, UT: Utah National Center For Voice And Speech.

Treder-Wolff, J. (2018) How Improv Changes Your Mind: It's Not What You Think, It's How. Accessed on 21/11/2019 at https://medium.com/@judetrederwolff/how-improv-changes-your-mind-its-not-what-you-think-its-how-ef12620c5a54

Verdolini Abbott, K. (2008) *Lessac-Madsen Resonant Voice Therapy*. San Diego, CA: Plural Publishing.

Vincent, B. (2018) *Transgender Health: A Practitioner's Guide to Binary and Non-Binary Trans Patient Care*. London: Jessica Kingsley Publishers.

Waller, N. and Penzell, S. (2019) 'A voice and communication program for transgender and gender diverse pediatric clients.' Presented at the European Professional Association of Transgender Health (EPATH), Rome, 11–13 April 2019.

Weir, K. (2012) 'The pain of social rejection.' *Monitor on Psychology, 43*(4), 50. Accessed on 21/11/2019 at www.apa.org/monitor/2012/04/rejection

White, M. (1997) 'Challenging the culture of consumption: rites of passage and communities of acknowledgment.' *Dulwich Centre Newsletter, 2 & 3*, 38–47.

White, M. (2007) *Maps of Narrative Practice*. New York: W.W. Norton & Co.

White, M. and Epston, D. (1990) *Narrative Means to Therapeutic Ends*. New York: W.W. Norton & Company.

Winslade, J. and Monk, G. (2007) *Narrative Counseling in Schools: Powerful and Brief*. Thousand Oaks, CA: Sage.

Wong, S.G.J. and Papp, V. (2018) 'Psychosocial and communicative impacts on the voice of trans men and transmasculine people: a global exploration.' Proceedings of the World Professional Association for Transgender Health (WPATH). Buenos Aires, Argentina: WPATH, 3–6 November 2018.

Wynn, N. (2019) Gender Critical: ContraPoints. Youtube video. Accessed on 21/11/2019 at https://youtu.be/1pTPuoGjQsI

Subject Index

Author Index